THE MERCENARY MAKEUP ARTIST

BREAKING INTO THE BUSINESS WITH STYLE

KAYLIN JOHNSON

The Mercenary Makeup Artist: Breaking into the Business with Style By Kaylin Johnson

© 2014 by Kaylin Johnson. All rights reserved.

First edition.

Visit our online directory at www.kaylinskit.com for links to resources mentioned in this book.

No part of this book may be reproduced in any written form, electronic form, recording, or photocopy without written permission of the author. The exception would be in the case of brief quotations embodied in critical articles or reviews and pages where permission is specifically granted by the author, Kaylin Johnson.

All brand names and product names mentioned in this book are trademarks, registered trademarks, and trade names of their respective holders. Mention of a company name does not constitute endorsement. The author is not associated with any product or vendor mentioned in this book, with the exception of affiliate relationships. The author uses affiliate links on her website, www.kaylinskit.com, for some companies mentioned in this book. However, she has attempted to provide unbiased information. Some companies mentioned in this book may have sent the author products free of charge for review purposes, but no additional compensation was accepted.

This book's purpose is to provide humorous and entertaining information on the topics covered. It is sold with the understanding that the author is not engaged in rendering legal, financial, accounting, business, medical, or any other professional advice or services. Although every precaution has been taken to verify the accuracy of the information contained herein, the author assumes no responsibility for any errors or omissions. No liability is assumed for damages that may result from the use of information contained within.

ISBN-13: 978-1-50082-663-5
ISBN-10: 1-50082-663-4

Cover Design: James, GoOnWrite.com
Cover Image: SL ADV/Shutterstock
Interior Design: Kaylin Johnson

Contents

Mission Briefing: The Mercenary Way 1

Mission 1: Intensive Training 6

Mission 2: Establish Credentials 13

Mission 3: Assemble Your Kit 17

Mission 4: Build Your Portfolio 35

Mission 5: Marketing and Networking 38

Mission 6: Taking Jobs 48

Mission 7: The Payout 59

Mission 8: Bridal Makeup for Mercenaries 64

Mission 9: Secret Techniques 77

Mission 10: Set Your Aim High 91

Dossier: Mercenary Resources 95

MISSION BRIEFING

The Mercenary Way

Stylish. Efficient. Professional. These are the hallmarks of a mercenary. They are also the makings of a great makeup artist. A professional arrives at the scene twenty minutes early, with hair perfectly styled and not a lash out of place. Her foundation is flawless, and her eyes are filled with confidence. She doesn't break a sweat as she wheels in her sleek kit, and then she whips out her makeup with superhuman speed. When the hair stylist flakes, she doesn't bat an eye—she has an array of tools in her trunk. In a matter of minutes, she transforms ordinary women into gorgeous models. When the shoot begins, she vanishes without a trace; her work is done. This is what it means to be a mercenary makeup artist. Do you think you have what it takes?

Why Mercenary

This book doesn't preach about inner beauty or creative dreams. I approach makeup from the perspective of a mercenary: simple, efficient, and effective. I'll cover every skill you'll need to know to survive out in the field, giving you the tools to become a mercenary makeup artist.

I won't waste your time with in-depth techniques—you'll need to master those on your own. Instead, this is a lean and mean guide to making money like a pro. I'll run you through career options, basic business principles, and getting jobs. I'll help you build a portfolio and assemble your ideal kit—but you're the one who will ultimately make it happen.

Finding Your Drive

You aren't going to become a professional overnight. It takes months of blood, sweat, and tears. If you're seeking fame or fortune, look elsewhere. Makeup is a service industry, and your livelihood will depend on pleasing your clients. If you are doing makeup because it sounds like a fun job or a good way to make money, this career isn't for you. The people who succeed are those who love makeup so much that they can't imagine doing anything else. They know what it means to be a mercenary and are prepared to accept even the lowliest of jobs in pursuit of their career.

Face the Facts

Mercenaries keep odd hours. Makeup artists have to be on set before actors or models—often with call times such as 4:30 a.m. Some makeup jobs require long hours or all-nighters. Makeup artists may sit around waiting for hours, then be asked to rush through dozens of looks. If you have a small child, school commitments, a demanding day job, or other obligations, think carefully about whether or not you can juggle them with makeup work.

Professionals must make sacrifices for a career in makeup. You'll volunteer your time and resources, travel across town through heavy traffic, and lose out on weekend time with your friends and family. When you have more experience, you can exercise some control over your hours, but mercenaries go where the work is, even if the hours are inconvenient.

CAREERS FOR MAKEUP ARTISTS

Very few artists work solely in film or other high-profile careers; those who do typically live in Los Angeles or New York. As a mercenary makeup artist, you need to master several niche fields. Diversify your skills to get consistent work. You might prefer applying zombie makeup over bridal makeup, but a mercenary can't afford to be picky if she wants to get paid.

Cosmetic salesperson – Hone your skills by starting out at a cosmetic counter or store. Some stores even offer training. If you're going to hold another job while pursuing your dream, this is about as close as it gets. Just make sure the company doesn't test on animals. You may be mercenary about makeup, but you don't want to promote cruelty. You can also take advantage of your employee discount to stock up your kit.

Face painter – No longer just about unicorns and cat whiskers, face painting can be a serious gig. Learn Day of the Dead face painting and other seasonal looks to get some cash on the side.

Bridal makeup artist – This field is a mercenary makeup artist's best friend. Brides are scattered across the nation and hold weddings throughout year. With regular work and large bridal parties, a makeup artist could almost make a living off this trade alone. If you haven't built up the capital or the courage to leap into full-time artistry, wedding work can be done as a weekend side job.

Print/editorial makeup artist – From senior photos to fashion magazines, print media offers a variety of opportunities for makeup artists. Photography studios sometimes offer little more than gas and supply money, while high-paying print jobs are often reserved for the most talented makeup artists in the area. If you want to work in this field, be prepared for some stiff competition.

Film/TV makeup artist – This is one of the most notoriously difficult fields for a beginning artist. Be prepared to put in your time doing zombie makeup or applying fake blood for student films. If you do get on a set, expect to touch up featured extras. While a variety of cities produce commercials and student films, the top professionals are often based in L.A. and New York. Some projects may require travel for extended periods, and be prepared for call times at all hours of the day. Smart mercenaries learn a marketable skill such as special effects makeup to increase their chances of a career in film.

Costume makeup artist – Most visible at Halloween, these artists use face paint, spirit gum, and other products to create fantastical looks from fairies to zombies. Some costume looks can be self-taught, but get professional training if this is your passion. Mercenaries can make money around Halloween with costume makeup.

Special Effects (SFX) makeup artist – Similar to costume makeup artists, Special Effects artists generally handle monster makeup, dramatic aging, and other transformations. These skills usually require extensive training at a school or other academy. Some professionals also hold workshops for this niche field. Mercenaries may not want to dedicate the time to learn this specialized field unless it is their ultimate dream.

Cosmetic consultant – If you have the expertise, you can generate income by working as a consultant for a cosmetic company. These roles can take on a variety of forms, such as advice to companies, feedback on new or existing products, color recommendations, or answers to common questions. Consulting roles can be good for mercenaries who prefer jobs with flexible hours. However, this type of work may be inconsistent.

MISSION BRIEFING: OBJECTIVE SUMMARY

1. **Find your drive.** What makes you want to be a makeup artist? Is it strong enough to sustain you through the challenges to come?
2. **Make a commitment to makeup.** A professional career requires a huge investment of time and effort. Are you ready to make the necessary sacrifices for this goal?
3. **Determine the tools you need.** Put together a list of the skills you'll need to make money like a mercenary. Which makeup jobs will be available in your area? Focus on marketable skills.

MISSION 1

INTENSIVE TRAINING

One of the first steps to becoming adept in any field is to humbly seek knowledge. Unlike many occupations, makeup artists can be self-taught. Yet this isn't always the simplest or most efficient method. Beauty school may be a good fit for some, despite the higher cost. Assess the benefits and trade-offs to find out which educational method is the most effective way to reach your goals.

BEAUTY SCHOOL BENEFITS

Getting a cosmetology or esthetician license. Makeup artists who are licensed cosmetologists and estheticians are qualified to do more than makeup. Licenses vary between states and countries, but cosmetologists can usually work with hair and estheticians can give facials. This opens up more possibilities for employment—ideal for mercenaries. Also, makeup artists typically need a license to work in a salon. Check your national, state, county, and city requirements to see if a license is required to practice makeup work.

Many cosmetic companies offer discounts to students and/or graduates. Even though classes may be expensive, you will usually qualify for discounts when building your kit. A cosmetology license is also a very easy way to qualify for almost every makeup artist discount available. Self-taught artists must provide proof of work, such as tear sheets or letters of employment to become eligible for the same discount.

Structured classes provide a focus. It's easy to become overwhelmed when you set out to master dozens of new makeup skills. An academic program provides structure and creates a financial commitment to learning. Mandatory practice hours translate directly into experience.

Cosmetology licenses incorporate a variety of skills, such as hair styling and nail care. Combination hair/makeup professionals are in high demand, especially for independent films and other smaller productions. A professional can easily double her income on a bridal job if she offers hair styling as well.

Beauty School Trade-Offs

Tuition is expensive. No matter how you pay for it, accredited programs typically cost thousands of dollars. A self-taught mercenary could purchase and maintain an entire professional kit for much less.

Makeup instruction may be limited, and taught out of a textbook. Many beauty schools focus on hair styling, waxing, or other techniques and offer little instruction in makeup. Also, professional makeup artists often earn a higher salary working in the field, so it is unlikely that you will find the world's top makeup artists teaching at a typical beauty school. There are some exceptions to this, such as the prestigious Make-up Designory in Hollywood, California. A mercenary could master the skills she needs on her own schedule if she's focused.

Schools may be far away or classes may be hard to fit into your schedule. The structure of an academic program can also be a problem for people with limited time. A school could also be hours away, and most of us can't get airlifted to class. Self-taught mercenaries can learn from their homes or become an apprentice, working around other commitments.

KNOW YOURSELF

A professional knows the path to success is defined by clear goals. Whether you're teaching yourself or following a course, keep laser-focused to get the most efficient training. Here are some questions to get you started:

1. What is my drive for becoming a mercenary makeup artist?
2. How do I define "professional makeup artist"?
3. Which types of paying opportunities are available in my city?
4. Which field(s) of makeup artistry do I need to master?
5. Would I consider moving to pursue this career? If so, where?
6. Do I want to be a makeup artist on the side or full-time?
7. How much can I afford to invest in this career?

A mercenary's goals must be realistic. If you're strapped for cash, watch free tutorial videos on YouTube and try out new techniques using drugstore makeup. Or work a part-time job to put yourself through school. Success is only possible if you're driven toward your goals.

The Self-Taught Mercenary

A motivated mercenary can teach herself a variety of skills, but only with diligence and patience. Few people will pay you to learn. Jobs at cosmetic counters and paid assistant work require at least a base level of knowledge. Start by mastering half a dozen distinct looks. If you plan to attend beauty school, supplement your coursework with additional self-taught skills.

Watch tutorial videos on sites such as YouTube. Find videos by professional makeup lines such as Jane Iredale, Scott Barnes, and MAC. There are also some decent videos by independent artists, such as Kandee Johnson and Michelle Phan. Mercenaries must be discriminating and seek out world-class mentors.

Seek out great texts. Study application techniques from books such as *Face Forward, Making Faces, The Bobby Brown Makeup Manual, Makeup Makeovers,* or *About Face.* Don't be surprised if you find conflicting information; artists have their own individual styles. A resourceful mercenary should experiment to see what works best for her. Books on color theory are also useful.

Buy a large palette of eye shadows. A colorful box of shadows is a handy tool for a mercenary's experiments. I keep a shadow set by budget brand NYX in my kit in case a client asks for an unusual color. Budget brands tend to go on more sheer, so apply them wet (also called "foiled") for a more dramatic look.

Vary your everyday makeup. Challenge yourself to try one completely new makeup look each week or even daily. A professional knows what works for her face and what doesn't. Recreate looks from magazines, ads, movies, or books. Be bold and make mistakes; it's better to make a mess of your own face than a client's.

Practice applying makeup on friends and family. Get a friend to bring over her makeup and brushes. Challenge yourself to create new looks from the resources you are given. Remember not to share makeup unless following proper sanitization practices. Invest in sanitizing products such as Beauty So Clean sanitizing mist and sanitizing wipes, as well as some disposable makeup sponges and a basic set of brushes. These will be indispensible tools during your mercenary career.

Once you've started gaining some confidence in your skills, move on to Mission 4: Build Your Portfolio.

BEAUTY SCHOOL SELECTION

When selecting a beauty school, a mercenary must be discerning. Look for schools that offer licenses as part of the program. If you are in the U.S., check for accreditation by the NACCAS (National Accrediting Commission of Career Arts and Sciences). Many other countries offer certification through similar organizations, such as Habia in the U.K. Examples of accredited schools in the U.S. include the Aveda Institute, Baldwin Beauty School, or Paul Mitchell – The School. Take a tour and drill your guide with questions. If you're going to be dropping thousands, make sure the school fits your specific needs.

Sample questions:

1. What does a typical day look like for a student at your school?
2. Are classes available during the day, evenings, or both?
3. How long does it take to complete the program?
4. What skills will I learn during the course of the program?
5. Does the program include license preparation work and any applicable testing fees?
6. How much does the program cost (including tuition and fees)?
7. What options are available for financial aid?
8. Are start dates available year round or only during select times each year?
9. How much hands-on experience do students get?
10. What types of careers do students pursue after graduation?
11. What type of assistance does the school provide for job placement upon graduation?
12. Is makeup coursework offered?

With the exception of a few schools, such as the Make-up Designory, most schools will offer coursework in two main fields:

Cosmetology – This type of program typically emphasizes salon skills related to hair. Programs will often offer courses in haircutting, hairstyling, and hair coloring, as well as nail technology and some makeup application.

Esthetics – Coursework for estheticians generally focuses on skin care. While programs differ between schools, you can expect to learn skills such as facial massage, aromatherapy, facial treatments, hair removal, lash and brow tinting, and more. Some makeup work is often included.

BE WARY

A professional always watches her back. If a program sounds too good to be true, it probably is. There are dozens of "schools" online that will sell you makeup instruction and a full kit. Don't expect them to offer the same benefits as an accredited program; there is often no license, professional supervision, or job placement assistance. If beauty school isn't an option for you, consider self-teaching and building your own custom kit, even if it is more expensive in the long run. You'll have the option of choosing your teachers and hand-selecting each item in your kit, which is invaluable for a mercenary.

MISSION 1: OBJECTIVE SUMMARY

1. **Choose your path.** Weigh the benefits and trade-offs of attending beauty school. Determine whether you want to attend school or if self-teaching is for you.
2. **If you're pursuing beauty school, find out how to enroll.** Research schools in your area. Visit the campuses and begin the admissions process.
3. **If you're planning to teach yourself, start today.** Watch a video tutorial, research books on makeup, or make a pledge to try one new look each week. Invite a friend over for a makeover and photo session.

MISSION 2

Establish Credentials

You should now know enough to be dangerous. An eager mercenary might want to jump straight into the field—but that could be deadly. Even a cosmetology license isn't enough. Before you accept a single penny, you'll want to make your business is official. Arm yourself with licenses and registrations from any applicable government institutions. Get your papers in order now and you'll see immediate benefits. You'll be able to make a website with your official business name, or start collecting receipts for tax-deductible business expenses.

Know Your Enemy

Don't go into the field flying blind. Whether you're a seasoned entrepreneur or starting from scratch, read up on business and marketing skills. Rudimentary mercenary texts include *The 4-Hour Workweek* and *The $100 Startup*, which help you set clear goals and cover basic marketing principles. For advanced mercenaries, try books such as *The 22 Immutable Laws of Marketing* or *NOLO's Small Business Start-Up Kit*.

A mercenary should also utilize local resources. SCORE offers free advice for small businesses. Look for local Meetup groups, community college courses on entrepreneurship, or events targeted toward small business owners. Groups for women in business often host events and some of these opportunities are open to men as well. Follow these steps to start to build a network of professionals.

D.B.A.s, Licenses, and Other Forms

A successful mercenary is an expert in her field, and business regulations are no exception. Before you accept payment from any client, check with your local city, county, and state institutions regarding any necessary forms and requirements. If you work under a pseudonym or business name in the U.S., you'll often be required to file a D.B.A. (Doing Business As) form. (Just don't put "mercenary" in the occupation field.) Makeup artists are typically considered sole proprietors, especially if they do freelance bridal makeup work with clients. Also check your national, state, and local requirements regarding any licenses required to work in makeup. In the U.S., some states have no requirements, but others do—especially in certain situations, such as salon settings. Call around and get some answers; online sources can be unreliable.

Makeup Artist Licenses

At the time of this writing, most states don't offer licenses for makeup artistry. However, if you plan to apply makeup in a salon, you will typically need a license in a field such as cosmetology. Check your national, state, and local requirements to make sure you are allowed to accept money for makeup work. Be prepared to answer questions such as how and where you plan to apply makeup. Also, selling makeup application services may not trigger sales tax requirements, but you might need a sales tax permit if you plan to sell cosmetics or other products.

Taxes

Even a professional can't be an expert in every field, so I urge you to consult an accountant regarding any tax questions. When a client writes you a check or pays you cash, you are still responsible for paying taxes on your earnings. An accountant can help you determine how much to file (and when), as well as provide information on tax-deductible expenses. Examples of deductible expenses might include makeup for your kit, mileage for makeup work, and other job-related expenses. Keep careful records and save receipts from any purchases you plan to claim as deductions. Also be wary of tax consequences of bartering. In some countries and states, goods such as photos can be considered taxable if you bartered your services with a photographer.

Some counties may also require you to charge sales tax, particularly if you plan to sell any products along with your services (such as skin care products or wholesale makeup). Your local county should be able to provide information on sales and use tax permits and requirements. Check these requirements before commencing paid work to avoid any potential fines.

Finances

A resourceful mercenary can fund her own business. If you don't attend beauty school, the biggest investment will be your makeup kit. Professional kits can run anywhere from $500 to $5000 and up. Consider opening a separate bank account for your business or making business purchases on a dedicated credit card. This helps keep business expenses separate from your personal expenses, which can simplify your tax records. As with all financial matters, consult an accountant or tax advisor for more information.

INSURANCE, WAIVERS, AND CONTRACTS

In the U.S., a professional can register her business as an LLC to keep her personal assets separate from her business. Consult a professional at SCORE or elsewhere for more information on the right type of business for your needs. Insurance can be purchased in most countries if liability is a concern.

A professional has her clients sign a combination contract and waiver before any application. This is my preferred method. I use one simple document to ensure any known allergies are disclosed, costs are clearly stated, and a waiver is in place. See Mission 8: Bridal Makeup for Mercenaries for more information on contracts.

MISSION 2: OBJECTIVE SUMMARY

1. **Learn how to start a small business.** Read books on entrepreneurship or talk to veteran business owners. Applying cosmetics is only a small part of a successful mercenary's career.
2. **Make it official.** If you plan to start your business under any name other than your own, register it with any applicable government agencies. Get your forms in order and determine whether you'll need to make special arrangements for business-related finances.
3. **Ask the tough questions.** Find out how to handle tax and liability concerns. Speak to accountants, lawyers, or other professionals who are qualified to answer your questions.

MISSION 3

ASSEMBLE YOUR KIT

A makeup artist's kit is her partner in the field. A well-stocked kit lets you create any type of look on any client, regardless of age, skin tone, or skin condition. It takes time and money to create the perfect kit, but you will learn to love it like a trusty sidearm. I depend on my kit to stay organized and on time. Keep essentials in stock and you might just be the unsung hero of a photo shoot.

Funding a Kit

A mercenary doesn't start out with a fully-stocked weapons locker, so you shouldn't expect to begin your career with a complete makeup kit. Pros need makeup suitable for any skin tone, but many artists start with a more limited range of colors. Just as a mercenary selects the right weapon for the job, you can use budget brands on your volunteer shoots. If you're worried about the quality, remember that affordable brands such as E.L.F. are found in pro kits.

Maintaining a Kit

Weapons require regular cleaning, and your kit requires vigilant maintenance. Liquid foundations, whether $8 or $50, often last only 6-12 months. Lip products, liquids, and creams might last a year or two, but even powders are typically replaced after 2-3 years. You might not think it's a big deal to use turquoise eye shadow from high school, but it's unprofessional—and often unsafe—to use expired products on your clients. They are relying on you to use only clean, sanitized makeup; your job and their health are on the line. The more you work, the more you'll see which products you use most. This should be what guides your future investments. I like to splurge on liquid foundations in lighter skin tones and a high-quality set of neutral eye shadows, but each artist's needs will be different.

For more on cosmetic expiration dates, see Mission 9: Secret Techniques.

Packing Tips

Once you have a kit, it's time to pack it like a mercenary—using a simple and efficient method. Group similar items together, based on makeup application stages. For example, dedicate one compartment for "face prep" supplies (witch hazel, primers, lip balm), another for base layers (foundation, concealer, powders), one for eye products, one for lip products, etc. Your needs may vary, so find a system that works for you. Remember, it's unprofessional to constantly hunt for supplies and keep your clients waiting.

Also remember that at many mercenary jobs, you will have to unpack and repack quickly. You'll often have little control over the location or the amount of space available. Consolidate your supplies. Think about what you can easily carry in one trip; returning to your car could mean leaving hundreds or thousands of dollars in makeup unattended. While most shoots are fairly secure, vigilance is key to keep your supplies from disappearing (particularly at unpaid gigs). I don't lock my kit, but I do keep my supplies contained and attended to discourage theft.

Just like a weapon, your kit needs to be handled with care. During hot summers and frigid winters, don't leave your kit in your car. Bring sensitive cosmetics such as foundations and creams inside with you, at the very least. If you travel by plane with your kit, be sure to pack it accordingly; bottles can leak (or worse) and pressed powders can break. You can lose valuable cosmetics this way.

If you're not sure what to bring for a job, pack for contingencies. When working volunteer shoots, I keep a duffel bag in my trunk with a hair dryer, hot rollers, curling iron, and other hair supplies. Hair stylists have stood me up on multiple occasions, so my hair tools have come in handy. I also keep a bag packed with specialty makeup, such as face paints, a big eye shadow palette, and spirit gum. I leave them at home for bridal jobs, but I've dug into that bag on more than one occasion for photo shoots with unpredictable needs.

Consolidating Your Kit

Mercenaries depend on efficiency. Individual lids and other obstructions can cost you valuable time. A professional consolidates her kit to travel light and stay on schedule.

Consolidate your pressed powder products by assembling them in a custom palette such as the Z palette. Cosmetics such as eye shadows, blushes, and bronzers can often be removed from their original packaging (a.k.a. de-potted) and combined in a magnetic palette. I carry two large palettes: one for my favorite eye shadows, and another with blush, bronzer, highlighter, and metallic eye shadows.

There are other ways to reduce the size and bulk of your kit. Carry multitasking products, such as neutral eye shadows, that double as brow powders. Bring travel-size versions of your larger liquids and moisturizers (purchase empty travel-sized containers and spray bottles). Take small amounts of other items, such as a stack of 25 tissues instead of a whole box. Use clear plastic bags to group similar items, such as eyeliners or light foundations.

Selecting Your Makeup

Purchasing makeup for a professional kit is very different than buying cosmetics for personal use. Mercenary makeup artists need products that are long lasting, high quality, and often heavier than everyday cosmetics. There may be some overlap with your personal cosmetics and those in your kit, but understand that you must shop with photography, studio lighting, water resistance, and other factors in mind.

Cruelty-Free Makeup

Seek out cruelty-free cosmetics. Cruelty-free refers to products that aren't tested on animals. There are various certifications companies can obtain, and sources such as PETA (People for the Ethical Treatment of Animals) offer detailed information on this topic. Budget brands such as E.L.F., NYX and Physician's Formula don't test on animals, and many higher-end brands have also made the pledge.

A professional buys a large quantity of makeup, so her purchases carry greater weight than an average consumer. Also, makeup artists are often in a position to make recommendations. Clients constantly ask me about products I use, and I proudly inform them that they are cruelty-free. These products are rarely more expensive, so support companies that have pledged to treat animals with compassion.

Allergies and Sensitivities

A professional applies products on all skin types, and some of her clients may be struggling with skin conditions. Ask your clients about any known allergies before applying makeup and have them sign a waiver (see Draw Up Bridal Contracts in Mission 8 for more information). Regardless, if you can't confirm whether or not your makeup contains an allergen and a client is highly sensitive (perhaps to gluten or latex), it's best to avoid using the product.

To avoid potential allergens, choose the "sensitive skin" option, if available. Look for products that provide good performance but are gentle on your clients. Research product reviews and search the Environmental Working Group's Skin Deep database. Try out natural brands, which tend to be safer for your clients and gentler in the long run.

Foundations

A professional needs foundations to suit any skin tone. It isn't efficient or necessary to carry foundations in every shade. Buy colors that mix well together. You'll probably want to carry at least five shades. Start with the lightest shade and the darkest shade. Look for lines that offer foundations deep enough for the darkest skin tones—not just "tan." For mixing, you'll want a mix of warm and cool (yellowish and pinkish) tones, along with a neutral. It's also good to have a tan/golden shade for mixing. Customize your shades to your needs. For example, if you work primarily with people of Caucasian, Hispanic, and Asian descent, carry more light shades and fewer darker shades.

Foundations come in many different forms, including powder, liquid, cream, mousse, and more. Liquids are my foundation of choice. They are very versatile, offer medium coverage (which can be built heavier) and look good on skin for almost any age range. If you also carry tinted powders (as setting powers), these can often double as foundation powders if you have a client who wouldn't look right in a liquid.

Also, avoid zinc as it can look white and/or pasty. This effect is common in some foundations with SPF. Sunscreens can also be potential allergens, so use only those with minimal to no SPF. If you are at an outdoor shoot, you can use a stand-alone sunscreen on your clients before applying foundation.

COLOR COSMETICS

When it comes to eye shadows, eyeliners, blushes, and lip products, mercenaries will need some variety. When choosing powder products, such as shadows and blushes, focus on matte products in versatile colors.

On almost every job, I use neutral eye shadows such as a creamy white, a neutral flesh tone, a soft gray-brown, and a dark coffee brown. You'll also want a pure black. Additional colors should be added based on what looks best on the largest number of your clients. Consider adding a light and dark set of colors such as forest green, sapphire blue, or plum. Gold and silver can also be useful. Wild colors such as bright yellows, vibrant oranges, and electric blues might be better off carried as part of a large, affordable palette—unless you specialize in colorful makeup. I rarely use shimmery and glittery makeup, as it is less versatile and the glitter tends to migrate on the face throughout the day. If you don't have shadows and liners to cover brow colors, make sure you purchase them as well. Don't forget auburn and gray.

For blushes and lip products, mercenaries should get a range of hues. For blushes, I like to keep a bright pink, a coral, and a purplish hue. I mix them for a custom look. Lipstick should be applied under lip gloss (if at all). I typically carry a lipstick palette with a range of pinks and some deeper hues, as well as a red or two. The most popular lip glosses in my kit are a shimmery brown and a soft bubbly pink (great for brides). Clear gloss can also be useful, particularly if you like using lipsticks. Don't forget red and neutral lip liners as well. You might not use lip liner as part of your everyday routine, but a neutral shade looks natural and helps lip color last longer.

Waterproof Makeup

A seasoned mercenary knows that waterproof cosmetics aren't just for underwater shoots. Waterproof mascara,

for example, is an essential for bridal makeup—
particularly for mothers and brides. Tell brides to remove
it using eye makeup remover or olive oil (in a pinch). I
don't use it on all my clients, as waterproof makeup is
more likely to cause itchiness or other reactions.

For beach and pool shoots, a professional may invest in
additional waterproof cosmetics. There are waterproof
eyeliners and other dedicated products, but the main
qualification is whether or not a product is oil-based.
Looks for creamy formulas, such as cream blushes and
oil-based foundations. If you live in an area that is very
rainy or has high humidity, waterproof makeup might be
an essential part of your kit.

Building a Brush Collection

Makeup brushes are essential tools of the trade. Before
you drop hundreds on a fancy pre-packaged brush set,
try building your own. A professional-quality set can be
assembled for a lot less than you think.

Look for brushes with durable handles made from
materials such as sustainably-grown wood or bamboo.
The ferrule (the metal band covering the point where the
brush meets the handle) should be a quality metal, ideally
recycled. Buy brushes with synthetic bristles. They are
cruelty-free and often provide equal, if not better, results.
Look for brushes from brands such as EcoTools, Bdellium
Tools (offers a makeup artist discount), Alima Pure, and
Crown Brush.

Buy a spare of each of your favorite brushes. You'll be
able to work on two clients before having to clean your

brushes. If you're working from light to dark eye shadow colors, you can sometimes use the same brush for two different shades. However, one brush per shade may help achieve a cleaner look. If you find yourself in a brush bind, you can always use a spray brush cleaner for a quick color change.

For more information on the brushes I recommend, see the Kit Contents section below.

A Clean Kit

A professional doesn't skimp on sanitization. Clients pay for a safe, hygienic application. Your reputation and your clients' health depend on your vigilance—so don't let them down.

Before applying makeup, wash your hands. If a sink isn't convenient, use hand sanitizer. Apply in front of your clients to give them peace of mind. Wash or sanitize your hands between clients.

Although I consider myself a "green" makeup artist, I utilize disposable items for hygienic purposes. These include items such as tissues, cotton balls, cotton swabs, paper nut cups (for mixing foundations), mascara wands, and foundation sponges.

Sanitizing Makeup

Mercenaries know how to make a clean getaway, and that means learning how to safely sanitize all cosmetics. To sanitize powders, apply a sanitizing spray such as Beauty So Clean over any powders used. Set powders aside and spray them together at the end of an application, or spray as you go. For eyeliners and lip liners, rub them over a sanitizing wipe such as Beauty So Clean wipes before sharpening (sharpen between each application).

The other way to keep your products clean is to properly dispense them as you go. Put foundation into a mini paper cup before mixing; never touch the pump or lip of the bottle to the foundation you've already dispensed. For cream concealers, lip balms, and lipsticks, swipe some onto a metal palette using the clean end of a makeup brush or a clean plastic spatula. Then apply from the palette. If you need more of a particular product, use another clean brush or spatula to swipe the product on a clean portion of the palette. This may seem tedious, but your clients' health is worth it. For maximum efficiency, choose products that are easy to dispense, such as squeezable lip glosses (instead of tubes with wand applicators).

One final option for sanitizing is a U.V. wand. They are often used in hospitals and other settings to kill germs and bacteria on the spot. It's ruthless but effective—a fitting tool for a mercenary.

CLEANING BRUSHES
When on a job, clean brushes with a quality spray brush cleaner. Spray onto a tissue and swipe the brush over the damp area until no pigment remains. Liquid brushes can be soaked in makeup remover (I use a small ceramic pot). Dry with a clean tissue. When making a quick getaway, wrap dirty brushes in a tissue.

When you arrive back at base, thoroughly wash any brushes you've used. Mix antibacterial dish soap with a bit of olive oil. Swirl the brush in the mixture and then rinse with warm water until the water runs clear. Repeat if necessary. Dry brushes by placing them at an angle so the tip is facing downwards on a lint-free cloth. This is especially important; water in the ferrule can loosen the glue and shorten the lifespan of a brush. Brush Guards (fitted brush sleeves) and special paintbrush holders can allow brushes to be dried with the tip directly down. These products may extend the longevity of your brushes and keep the bristles looking like new. However, it can be an investment to outfit an entire kits' worth of brushes with the guards or buy a sufficient number of specialty dryers.

Makeup Artist Discounts

If you're a cosmetology student or have a few credits to your name, you may qualify for some discounts on cosmetics. These deals are often known as professional discounts, pro artist programs or MUA (makeup artist) discounts. Some companies are quite generous, offering 40% or more off products, but most are in the 15-25% range. Some lines may also offer trial or sample sizes to artists, which can be a great way to get a variety of colors in a small, affordable package.

When you're just starting out, it can be tough to meet the requirements for discounts, but it's worth looking at your favorite cosmetic companies to see what you'll need to qualify. Typical requirements are agency credentials; credits in TV, film, or print; a cosmetology license; or proof of student status. Some companies accept a website, business card, or a letter of reference, but this is more rare.

Keep in mind that some makeup companies also offer discounts for actresses, models, and dancers. If you have experience in one of those fields, you may be able to meet the requirements through that route. Just read the terms and conditions carefully.

If you're interested in a cosmetic line that doesn't publicize a makeup artist discount, contact them directly. Many discounts are unpublished. If none are available, sometimes a company will mention other pathways to discounts, such as an email list or an affiliate program.

BRAND RECOMMENDATIONS

Below is a list of brands with products suitable for a professional. Many of these are brands are in my kit. These brands are available in the U.S.; local and international availability may vary. Each line has its strengths, so test products before you buy or purchase from a retail store that allows returns of opened items, such as Sephora or CVS.

100% Pure, Afterglow Cosmetics (MUA Discount), Alima Pure, Beauty Without Cruelty, DeVita, Ecco Bella, Eyes Lips Face (E.L.F.), Gabriel Cosmetics/Zuzu Luxe (MUA Discount), Glo Minerals, Jane Iredale (MUA Discount), Josie Maran, Korres (MUA Discount), Kryolan (MUA Discount), Mehron, NVEY Eco, NYX (MUA Discount), Physician's Formula, Tarte Cosmetics, Urban Decay (MUA Discount)

Note: "MUA Discount" refers to brands which offer a makeup artist discount (see Makeup Artist Discounts above).

For links, please see Dossier: Mercenary Resources or go to www.kaylinskit.com.

KIT OPTIONS

Just as explosives need to be packed with care, a mercenary's makeup requires a special case or bag. A stylish case is a bonus, but the real measure of a makeup kit is its practicality. Look for an option with wheels, one light enough to lift (even with twenty or more pounds of cosmetics), and organizational compartments. The two most popular options are below:

Train cases – This is your typical makeup artist kit. They are essentially boxy, hard-sided suitcases that prop open and have multiple compartments. A mercenary on a budget can buy her first case at a hardware store; look for tool boxes or bags, ideally with wheels. Prices and styles will vary.

ZUCA bags – The ZUCA pro is my ideal mercenary kit. It comes with several stackable zippered mesh bags to keep a kit organized. It also has an aluminum alloy frame that serves as a seat for you or any client up to 300 lbs. This is particularly useful in remote locations and busy airports. The bag fits into most overhead bins and is light enough to lift (if packed properly). ZUCA pros can cost around $300, but the company also offers less expensive bags with some of the same features.

Kit Contents

A mercenary's makeup needs will vary greatly. An SFX makeup artist requires a different set of supplies than a bridal makeup artist. The list below is for the everyday mercenary, who will be working primarily on bridal, editorial, and commercial shoots. I have also listed optional add-ons for mercenaries with different specialties or the financial resources to build a bigger kit. I only pack the items listed in Beyond the Basics if a job requires them.

For a kit checklist, go to www.kaylinskit.com.

Cosmetics and Related Items

Prepping the Face – Makeup remover towelettes (individually wrapped), eye makeup remover, witch hazel (toner), moisturizer for sensitive skin, liquid primer, unscented lip balm

Face/Base layer – Liquid foundations (usually at least five colors ranging from lightest to darkest, with colors in between to adjust red and yellow tones when mixed), a palette of cream concealers and/or correctors in a range of colors (again lightest, darkest, and correctors in colors such as peach, yellow, and/or green), setting powder (one in a universal shade and at least 3-5 tinted shades)

Face/Cheeks – Blush (at least 3 colors, such as a pink, a coral, and a purplish hue), bronzer (at least two to accommodate different skin tones; certain eye shadows can double as bronzers), highlighter (often a sheer, shimmery eye shadow can double as a highlighter)

Eyes – Eye shadow primer, pressed powder eye shadow (quality matte neutrals; popular colors such as blue, purple, and green in dark/light sets; fun colors and metallics in a big, cheap palette), eyeliner (pencils in black and brown—adding in other colors later—and ideally a black cream as well), mascara (waterproof and regular), false eyelashes (strips and/or individual), eyelash glue, eyelash glue remover

Brows – Brow powder and pencils for blonde, medium brown, dark brown, auburn, gray, and black (brow powders and pencils may double as eye shadows and eyeliners if shades are matte)

Lips – Lip liner (2-3 neutral shades and a true red), lip gloss (clear and shades such as brown, peach, pink, and red), tinted lip balm, lipstick (a palette, black, and 1-2 reds)

Finishing touches – Makeup setting spray

ACCESSORIES

Brushes – Slick foundation brushes (at least 2), slick concealer brushes (2), eye shadow crease brushes (2), eye shadow lid brushes (2), eye shadow smudge brushes (2), small angle liner brushes (at least 2; these double as a brow brushes), a lash and brow groomer, a dense blush brush, a flat-topped bronzer brush, a fan brush (for removing stray powder), kabuki powder brushes (2), a brow spoolie (looks like a long mascara wand), slick mini lip brushes (6)

Disposable items – Tissues, cotton balls, cotton swabs, foundation sponges, paper nut cups (for mixing foundations), foundation sponges, plastic spatulas, mascara wands

Sanitization – Beauty So Clean spray (in a travel bottle), Beauty So Clean wipes, brush cleaner (in a travel bottle), hand sanitizer

Courtesy items – Gum or mints (for you and/or clients), bottled water

Nails – Nail polish in 1-2 versatile colors, nail file, nail clippers

Hair – Comb, brush, hair clips (for pinning client hair back), hair elastics, bobby pins, hair spray

Grooming – Tweezers, battery-operated personal groomer (for shaving eyebrows and other facial hair), small scissors (for trimming false lashes)

Business items – Business cards, pens (at least 3), Sharpie (to label water bottles), sticky notes, face charts

"Just in case" items – Eye drops, over-the-counter medications for allergies or headaches, band-aids, first aid kit, sewing kit, stain remover pen, double-sided tape, clothespins

Miscellaneous – Metal makeup palette, hand mirror (for showing client final look), small ceramic pot (for soaking slick brushes in makeup remover), travel-sized water spray bottle (for wetting brushes to create "foiled" looks), pencil sharpener (for sanitized liner pencils), heated eyelash curler (and extra batteries), unpetroleum jelly (as brow gel), straws (so clients don't mess up lip products), plastic shopping bag (with no holes; for trash)

Beyond the Basics
Specialty items – Bruise makeup palette, face paints (such as white for ghosts), face painting palette (looks like watercolors), spirit gum, spirit gum remover, fake blood, latex (or latex alternative if you or your clients are allergic)

Hair styling tools – Blow dryer (can also be used to soften hard pencils), curling iron(s), straightener, hot rollers, bobby pins in multiple colors, hair elastics in multiple colors

Airbrush – Airbrush, airbrush makeup

Miscellaneous – U.V. sanitizing wand, director's chair, folding table (to lay out your kit)

Mission 3: Objective Summary

1. **Determine your budget.** How much can you afford to spend on a makeup kit? Decide how you will fund your kit. Will you be making a large investment or do you plan to add a few items each month?
2. **Make a wish list.** Determine what resources you have available, and which items you'll need to purchase. Go to cosmetic stores and other retailers to test products before making a large purchase. See www.kaylinskit.com for a budgeting worksheet and a kit checklist.

3. **Build your first kit.** Purchase your first kit bag or case. Buy the items you'll use immediately, or fill it with all the essentials if you have a generous budget. Pack your kit and start developing your own organizational system.

MISSION 4

BUILD YOUR PORTFOLIO

Once your kit is armed and ready, it's time to start building your portfolio. A strong portfolio can help land you bridal jobs, commercial gigs, and other work. Use your training as a guide for the types of shoots you should pursue. Focus on what is commercially viable, not just what sounds fun.

TAKE THE FIRST PHOTOS

A professional documents her work. Take before and after shots of the looks you practice on friends and family. Bring your "clients" into natural light and snap a few digital pictures that include their head and the tops of their shoulders. Have them sign photo releases. These images will help aspiring photographers determine your abilities. The makeup doesn't have to be perfect, but stick with your strengths. Tasteful, everyday looks are easiest to master.

CONNECT WITH PHOTOGRAPHERS

Build a profile on a model/photographer networking site such as Model Mayhem. Post images of your best work. Be aware that many of these sites contain adult images and offer adult-oriented shoots. Search through photographers who are willing to "TFP" or "TFCD," which stands for "trade for prints" or "trade for CD." You want to find models and photographers who will volunteer their time to get images for portfolio building. Draw up a

TFP contract to ensure your photographer delivers images on time. See www.kayilnskit.com for a sample contract.

A beginning portfolio is unlikely to attract top photographers. Continue going to photo shoots and update your portfolio with higher quality images. Eventually, you'll be able to reach out to professional-level photographers.

Seek out photo shoots that cater to your goals, while still showing diversity. Whether or not you enjoy bridal work, seek out wedding looks. Arrange a shoot with models in wedding dresses (from a thrift store or their own wedding). Showcase your talents on people of varying ethnicities and genders. Clean, natural looks are great sellers, but don't be afraid to include one or two creative shots in your portfolio to demonstrate your range. If your experimental makeup looks don't turn out well, try again with a different creative team or expand your talents in another direction.

Seek Out a Mentor

Every master was once an apprentice. Search for successful artists in your area. Reach out to them, offering to assist for free with anything from cleaning brushes to applying foundation. Tell them you are just getting started in the industry and would love to observe them in action. You may find an artist who needs help with large weddings and other projects. Apprentice work may lead to paid assistant work in the future.

If a potential mentor is too busy, ask if they would be willing to answer some questions for you. Many artists want to help, provided you are respectful of their time and show a willingness to learn.

Review Your Portfolio

The transition to paid field work can be daunting. When I finally landed my first bridal job, the work was hardly consistent. Until you're at the point where your images stand up to other professional work in your area, it's a good idea to keep building your portfolio. Once you have confidence in your work, then it's time to start putting yourself on the market.

Mission 4: Objective Summary

1. **Take your initial photos.** Snap some shots of your early work. Whether your first makeovers are on friends, mothers, sisters, or boyfriends, document them carefully with before and after shots. This will serve as your very first portfolio.
2. **Reach out to other amateurs.** Connect with aspiring photographers and models on Model Mayhem or other networking sites. Start going to photo shoots and getting comfortable on set. Get familiar with the application process and working with clients.
3. **Collect a portfolio of great images.** It may take dozens of photo shoots to get one great image. Take your time to get a wide range of looks on a variety of models. Your portfolio should be 10-20 images or more of your best work.

MISSION 5

Marketing and Networking

An artist with professional-level images is ready to make her presence known. For maximum exposure, create a web presence while building a local network. Having an online presence will help establish trust with local clients, which is essential to getting paid work—particularly when you're new to the industry.

Create a Web Presence

Website

Even if you have a fantastic portfolio on a website like Model Mayhem, a personal website is much more professional. Mercenaries need to reach out to a broad audience, and a website allows brides, photographers, editors, and others to view your work and get a sense of you as a professional.

Include a portfolio of only professional-level images, showcasing the breadth of your talents on a variety of models. If you're looking to specialize in a niche market such as effects work, create a separate portfolio for that field (once you have several high-quality images to fill it). Add a short biography, a service list (posting rates is optional), and a contact page. Don't post your physical address or email (to avoid spam), but do include a contact form so clients can reach you.

An attractive website doesn't have to cost thousands. Tech-savvy mercenaries can create their own website for free on a site like Wix.com. Wix offers several attractive templates to modify to suit your needs. A professional should buy her own custom domain. If you're on a tighter budget, you can also create a website using a blogging platform such as Blogger or Wordpress, but it often takes more work to achieve the sleek presentation of paid or ad-driven services.

If you're not technically inclined, consider hiring someone to help build your website. A simple site is a bit of an investment, but don't pay thousands for features you don't need. Websites such as Elance and Wix can help you connect with web developers who can work within a modest budget.

Social Networking
While websites provide a long-term presence, social networking is a great way to remind people you are an active field operative. Choose 1-2 outlets, such as Facebook, Twitter, or Instagram. Create an account dedicated to your business. If you have permission from clients, post photos from the set. Offer weekly makeup tips or other interesting tidbits. Post frequently, but only as often as you can produce quality content. For example, I tend to post 1-2 times per week. Focus your efforts on helping others, rather than self-promotion. Tutorials, day-in-the-life posts, and pros tricks can provide fun and helpful information for your followers.

BLOGGING AND VIDEOS

For those who are skilled with words, a blog can be a great way to explore another aspect of the beauty industry. Blogs are typically based on niche hobbies. My blog, Kaylin's Kit, focuses on vegan and eco-friendly makeup. Some makeup artists share step-by-step tips, recreate popular looks, blog about jobs (with clients' permission), or review products. Your blog could be a combination of any or all of these, but keep a central focus to attract a loyal audience.

For those who are skilled with computers, YouTube videos are another option. Artists such as Michelle Phan and Kandee Johnson made a name for themselves using this method. Typically videos are step-by-step tutorials, makeup reviews, or behind-the-scenes features. While some people make a lot of money from YouTube and other video outlets, they are generally the exception to the rule. It can take over 10-20 hours to make each video, and considerations have to be taken for lighting, royalty-free music, costumes, and more. Videos aren't the best way to establish a local presence, but they could potentially lead to paid work down the line—perhaps from other sources.

If you choose to blog or make videos, be sure to post about them on social media to maximize your exposure.

OTHER OUTLETS

Mercenaries who are looking for exposure should register with websites such as Yelp and Google Places. Yelp allows clients to leave reviews, whether they are positive or negative. To get reviews, send thank-you emails to clients after successful jobs. Include a note such as "If you enjoyed your experience, please consider leaving a review on Yelp.com [insert link to your page here]. If you found our service unsatisfactory in any way, please let us know so we can correct the issue promptly."

If bridal makeup is a central part of your mercenary plan, there are also some wedding websites that will list makeup artists. Sites such as Wedding Wire offer paid and non-paid options to list your business. Many of these sites also include options for brides to review your business. Before investing in these services, consider carefully. A good mercenary never gets pressured into paying for services she doesn't need. It can be easy to drop hundreds or thousands before you've worked a single wedding.

Build Your Underground Network

While creating your portfolio, you have been building a network of local photographers, models, and other connections. However, your network shouldn't be limited to people with whom you've already worked. A professional actively seeks new clients.

Attending Bridal Shows

Your underground networking should be simple and efficient. Connect with a large number of professionals by attending local events such as bridal shows. While you can do this as a vendor, it's not nearly as efficient as attending as a normal "guest." For a nominal entry fee, some shows will let you walk the floor freely and connect with dozens of photographers, venues, and wedding planners. Just be sure to check the rules of the show so you don't get thrown out for soliciting. Vendors pay hundreds of dollars for tables at these events, and you want to give them the chance to make good use of their time in front of the brides. Never—NEVER—solicit brides directly at shows unless you've paid for a table.

When attending shows—whether as a vendor or as a guest—dress in business casual attire and wear flawless makeup. When approaching vendors, be sure to wait patiently for vendors to finish talking with any brides or couples. As a makeup artist, you are a business—not a potential customer. Smile and introduce yourself as a makeup artist. Give them a compliment and tell them that you are there to connect with other industry professionals. Ask if you can post a link to their services on your website. Offer them a postcard, business card, or flier (see below) so they can see your work. Collect the vendor's business card and write down their name if it isn't listed.

Don't hesitate to approach other makeup artists as well. Even mercenaries sometimes need to work in teams. Network with other artists so you can call on them if you get offered a job you can't handle alone. If an artist's work is good, you can also recommend them to brides when you're overbooked. Some makeup businesses have several artists on staff, and may be looking to add to their roster.

After the show, take all the vendor business cards you've collected and email every connection. Remind the vendor who you are and ask if you can to list their business on your website. If they agree, follow through and list them on your site. Add them to your contacts for the future.

Seek Out Other Markets

Resourceful mercenaries look for other ways to connect with local clients. While it may be tempting just to seek out work in your desired specialty, mercenaries understand that this is a competitive business. Cast a wide net for paid work if you want to work regularly.

Modeling – Check casting calls on sites such as Model Mayhem, and consider doing some unpaid work if you have the chance to work with a great team. Reach out to modeling agencies—if there are reputable agencies in your area (be wary of modeling schools that are also agencies). Seek out fashion shows in your area and connect with the organizers. Offer to help, and be prepared to do so—even if unpaid. There are often shows at bridal expos, charity fashion shows, mall events, and other opportunities that provide runway fashion makeup experience.

Commercial Photography – Connect with local photographers—particularly those who do headshots or bridal work. Look for photography open houses, workshops, or networking groups. Search for local magazines and reach out to their editors and photographers. Some may arrange a trade or volunteer shoot to have you prove your talent.

Film and Video – Look for crew calls for independent films and search for film community directories (such as local film commissions). Offer your services as an unpaid assistant or intern. Mercenaries who can do some light effects makeup, such as zombies, aging, gore and blood, will find more opportunities. Reach out to film schools in your area to find work on student films. Be extra cautious of opportunities on Craigslist, as many may be adult in nature or generally suspect.

Other Opportunities – New businesses may need makeup work on photo shoots for clothing, accessories, and jewelry. Ask a bridal shop if you can leave some fliers or business cards; many have vendor bulletin boards. A resourceful mercenary will always keep an eye out for local events that may require makeup work. Ballets, plays, music festivals, and film festivals can all be great places to gain experience.

Business Cards and Fliers

Strive to achieve maximum effectiveness with the least effort. Make a smart investment in a quality business card. If you have a stylish card, people will take you seriously—no matter how much experience you have. A great business card leaves a professional impression, so back it up with great work on the job as well.

You have probably seen advertisements for free business cards, or wondered about printing your own cards. Don't be fooled by these poor investments. The quality is often poor and the designs can easily look dated.

Mercenaries on a budget can use Moo.com. They offer regular-sized cards or mini cards (half size). Print your best portfolio image on one side, and another great picture on the reverse (along with your contact info). Or use Moo's template designs to make a set. Moo cards are printed on quality paper and get compliments.

For those with a little more to spend, Taste of Ink is a good option. Taste of Ink offers custom designs and details like embossing. Even a basic card from a company like Taste of Ink makes a great impression.

A professional should also create a postcard for bridal shows. Put your best bridal image on the front, and another on the back. Include your contact information and explain that you specialize in bridal makeup. Print the postcards at a professional printer (online or otherwise). Use a glossy finish for a professional look. Print your rates separately on a half-sheet or full sheet of paper. If you're going to use half-sheets, cut them with exacting precision. Otherwise, use a full sheet.

When printing materials, think like a mercenary. Conserve resources by choosing recycled paper and only printing what you need. In your first year, you will likely hand out no more than 50 postcards, and fewer than 200 business cards. Don't be fooled into printing 1,000; it isn't efficient or cost-effective.

Networking Tips

No matter how large or small your underground network may be, keep it organized with mercenary efficiency. Keep a separate address book (digital or physical) with your business contacts. If you have a good experience with a photographer, add them. If you meet a great makeup artist on a volunteer gig, list them as well. Skilled makeup artists can assist you with large parties; recommend them if you have to refuse a job.

Some contacts like to connect through social networking sites such as LinkedIn. Others may want to add you on Facebook or other sites, which is why it's good to have a separate account or profile for your business. A professional keeps her business separated from her personal life.

If you want to keep up with your contacts, send holiday or New Year's cards. Websites such as Punchbowl.com offer digital cards, which only require an email addresses. Send something memorable—perhaps a snapshot of some of your more artistic work. A professional makes a lasting impact without being annoying or offensive.

When interacting with other businesses, offer an incentive for helping you. List the business on your website or offer a special deal for their customers. Wear flawless makeup when you meet with vendors. Dress professionally and exude confidence. For more tips, check out books such as *How to Win Friends and Influence People*.

Even the best marksmen don't have perfect aim, so don't be discouraged if your networking isn't 100% successful. People get busy, change careers, and generally have their own problems. Diversify your contacts so you are less dependent on any single opportunity or revenue stream. This strategy gives you a better chance of regular income.

Mission 5: Objective Summary

1. **Build a website.** Present your portfolio on a sleek online website. Provide a place for clients to easily find out more about your services. If you aren't tech-

savvy, find someone with the skills to help you build an affordable and eye-catching site.
2. **Find other ways to connect online.** Register for social media websites or create a blog. Expand your online presence so your website doesn't get lost in cyberspace.
3. **Create a business card.** Visit a website such as Moo.com to design your business card. List your website and other relevant information. Choose a unique, eye-catching design.
4. **Attend a local networking event.** Go to a local bridal show and connect with industry professionals. Look for fashion shows, student films, photography workshops, and other events where you can gain experience and meet other professionals.

MISSION 6

TAKING JOBS

You've trained, practiced, and landed your first paying job. So what do you do when you get there? Confidence is half the battle. Follows these tips and you might just fool everyone into thinking you're already a seasoned professional.

ALWAYS BE PREPARED

A makeup job starts before you step in the door. A professional prepares ahead of time, so she can maximize her time on the set. You never know how much time you'll have to apply makeup, and the faster you can produce quality work, the better. It's best if you're the one waiting on photographers and models. Never—NEVER—be the one to hold up the shoot.

The number one way to prepare is to have a clean, well-stocked kit. Make sure your brushes are clean. I keep a tissue in my brush box, which I set out beneath my brushes on location. Review the list in Mission 3: Assemble Your Kit to make sure you've got the essentials and a few "just in case" items. Clothespins, band-aids, and hair styling tools can sometimes save the shoot.

When working with a bride or actor on more than one occasion, assemble a special plastic bag with their makeup. Keep a bag for each character in a film, or one for each member of the bridal party. If you can't separate items like eye shadows from a large palette, at least set aside foundation colors or other items.

Do your research. If you're doing a shoot with face paint, study up on creative looks in the medium. Practice on yourself or a friend first, if possible. If you're doing a pool shoot, test out your underwater makeup. Don't expect to learn everything on the set; study up ahead of time and arrive an expert.

Dress to Impress

A mercenary always looks the part, no matter how early or late the job. I typically wear a black blazer, a solid tee shirt, nice jeans, and ballet flats or low dress boots. Tie your hair back. Shower and wear either impeccable makeup or no makeup whatsoever. Don't forget deodorant. As you will be in close proximity to clients, use mints or gum. Don't wear perfume, as it could trigger allergies in your clients, which can ruin the entire job.

Arrive Early

Always arrive early to jobs. You can follow every other tip in this book, but if you can't be punctual, you will not survive as a makeup artist. Double-check the time of your job and put reminders wherever you will see them. Set multiple alarms, lay out your clothes the night before, or whatever else you need. If you can't make it to a shoot early, don't accept the job. Assume there will be traffic, construction, daycare issues, daylight savings, or any other complication and allow extra time for it.

If you arrive on time or later, you are late. Being late means you have failed the job. Professionals don't hold up shoots—they save them. Remember that you'll need time to set out your kit, wash your hands, eat a snack, etc. Plan to arrive at least 20 minutes early—10 at the absolute latest. It's always better to wait on the clients than to have them wait on you. If you aren't allowed to arrive early, wait in your car or hang out at a nearby coffee shop. Just remember to bring sensitive cosmetics inside if it's a particularly hot or cold day.

BE PRESENT

A professional leaves all her personal and emotional baggage at the door. If you are harried from traffic, take a few calming breaths before leaving your car. Your job isn't just to apply makeup; you also need to help anyone who sits in your chair feel more confident. A makeup artist must be of service to the client—so make good use of this time to help her day go better. Focus on the task before you, and clear your mind of unnecessary distractions.

KNOW YOUR PLACE

A professional knows she's not the focus of the shoot. Makeup artists are hired to make a bride feel beautiful, execute a photographer's vision, or sell a product. A mercenary must defer to the client and their vision. You might makes suggestions based on your expertise, but your primary job is to keep your clients satisfied. Some fashion photo shoots, for example, are all about breaking the established rules and using unconventional color combinations. Trust in the client's vision, and understand your role. A successful mercenary learns to find satisfaction in a job well done, rather than in uncompromising artistry.

Lend a Hand

Professional shoots and films often have production assistants and other staff dedicated to keeping the shoot running smoothly. This is rarely the case for the mercenary jobs you'll get at this stage in your career. You might be on a photo shoot with two different looks: a soft daytime look and a dramatic evening look. When the photographer is shooting the first look, you may have little to do. Instead of waiting around, offer to lend a hand while they are shooting the first look. Hold a light reflector for the photographer or adjust hair and clothing. Your assistance will improve the quality of the product and, by extension, your work.

Offer to Stand In

A professional knows that she can be more than just a makeup artist. If the hair stylist doesn't show, offer to do some light hair styling. You might not have time to do a full updo or other complicated look, but adding a few waves can greatly improve the final images. A diligent mercenary checks state regulations regarding hair styling—particularly for paid work. Sometimes the models may have to be the ones to use the styling tools.

There's a chance you might be asked to model—either on the spot (due to a no-show) or at a later date. Whether or not you're comfortable in front of cameras, modeling can be a worthwhile experience. If a photographer asks you to model, trade for headshots or photos of you applying makeup. You can use these high-quality images on your website. This is another reason to arrive at shoots looking your best.

However, a professional knows where to set her boundaries. If you get offers for boudoir shoots or other risqué jobs, turn them down. Put your safety first, and your reputation next—you'll have plenty of opportunities to make contacts without jeopardizing both.

Advocate for Yourself

A successful mercenary watches her own back. Shoots can be intense and demand long hours. It can be tough to remember to eat and take breaks. Your client may put pressure on you to work quickly, so advocate for your needs. Take a bathroom break or eat a snack if you need it. Bring extra food in case a shoot runs late. Pack protein bars, fruit leathers, or trail mixes. Keep granola bars on hand—for you or the occasional starving client. Even if jobs claim to offer food, don't depend on it. Bring your own water and pack a few disposable bottles of water as well for clients.

If you're working in hot conditions, plan accordingly. Bring plenty of water. Carry a cooler for sensitive cosmetics like creams and liquids. Pack electrolyte powders or sports drinks. Dress in sun-reflective clothing, wear a wide-brimmed hat, and bring plenty of sunscreen.

If you're working in cold conditions, bring hand warmers, wear plenty of layers, and carry a thermos with a hot beverage. Wear fingerless gloves when applying makeup.

A professional never skimps on sanitizing—even when she's in a rush. Take the time to clean brushes between clients. If you're constantly falling behind because of brush cleaning, invest in a second set of brushes. If your feet are tired, bring a folding chair so you can sit. You don't have to lean over to apply makeup. Buy a director's chair to bring clients up to you.

Leave No Trace

When a professional leaves a shoot, her workspace is spotless. Makeup belongs on your client's face—not on clothes, countertops, or floors. It may seem simple, but it can be tricky in practice. Your kit is full of products designed to color and, in some cases, stain.

Leave the scene exactly as you found it. Check your kit for dirt and mud before rolling it indoors. Look for any pigments on makeup bags or trays before setting them out. Place tissues beneath your brushes. If your brushes are wet, pile on extra tissues. Put makeup back in its proper place as you work. Don't set it on a counter or other workspace you don't own—unless it is lined with tissues. Makeup containers in a kit tend to pick up residue and pigments which can easily stain.

Your clients pay a premium for precision, so don't leave makeup on their clothes or hair. Keep hair off a client's face using hair clips (unless a hair stylist tells you otherwise). Most clips are gentle enough not to crease hair. If you need to apply makeup near clothes, costumes, or accessories, stuff tissues around collars or sleeves. Place tissues carefully; even a drop of foundation could disrupt a shoot. A professional keeps a stain remover pen in her kit, but she is never the cause of a stain.

A professional also takes out her own trash. Carry a plastic shopping bag for dirty tissues, disposable mascara wands, sanitizing wipes, and any other garbage. Take it back to base and empty it in your personal garbage. Many locations will have trash cans on hand, but they might not be convenient. It's rarely a good idea to use these trash cans, especially if you're borrowing someone's home as a photo shoot location.

Defer to Clients and Mentors

Know how and when to follow orders. Typically there will be one person in charge who holds the creative vision. Listen to this person and follow their advice. If you don't agree with what another artist is doing, hold your tongue. Unless you have specifically been placed in charge of that artist, it's not your responsibility to tell them how to do their job. Feel free to give compliments, however, if they are due. Working with other artists can be a great way to pick up techniques, hear product recommendations, and build a network of contacts.

If you are working as an assistant beneath a more senior makeup artist, or if he is your boss or mentor, defer to him for how to behave on set. If he asks you to only apply foundation, do it. If he wants to teach you a new skill, listen carefully. If you don't understand an instruction, ask for clarification. There is no harm in asking for help—especially when his name is on the line.

Some artists are also very particular about networking on jobs. If you are hired as a representative of a company or as someone's assistant, ask ahead of time how to handle a request for business cards. Some people believe that the person who booked the job is the one who gets credit, and those who help them are only there as part of that business. Others consider you an independent artist, so they might not mind if you hand out your own business cards.

Handle Disagreements Gracefully

Handle even the most challenging situations with grace. For large-scale events, a team of artists often works toward one unified goal. You may apply someone's entire look, but don't be surprised if another artist changes your look to suit the organizer's updated vision. Changes like this happen all the time, so give the other makeup artists the benefit of the doubt.

However, a professional may sometimes need to speak up. I was once on a Victorian-era shoot where the organizer wanted a very soft look. I did a model's makeup and had it approved by the organizer. A few minutes later, the model reappeared wearing dark, heavy eyeliner applied in a wobbly line. I took the organizer aside and privately mentioned that the model had made additions to her look after we'd approved it. The organizer immediately understood and decided to never work with that model again—for that and several other reasons.

While I received the benefit of the doubt in that situation, it won't always be the case. If you disagree with someone, it's usually best to hold your tongue. If you think your reputation may be on the line because of someone else's actions, then you may want to privately discuss it with the person in charge. The beauty industry can be a very small field and makeup is a subjective art. A smart mercenary knows when to swallow her pride to avoid making enemies.

Leave When Asked

A makeup artist may be asked to stay on for the shoot to touch up lipstick and powder, but her high hourly rates make this a rare occurrence. When your work is done, the best thing you can do is get out of the way. Pack up your kit as quickly as possible. Handle brush cleaning and kit reorganization at home. However, if the client offers to let you stick around and you want to, feel free to do so.

Put Safety First

Before attending a job, a smart mercenary will research her client. Make sure they are legitimate—especially if it is a photographer with a home studio. A photographer who shoots nudes isn't necessarily disreputable, but review their images to see if you want to be connected with their work. I focused on fully-clothed shoots, as I felt they would be most versatile in my portfolio.

Some photographers will also allow you to have an "escort" for the shoot, such as friend, significant other, or parent. Certain professionals look down on bringing escorts, but I tend to be wary of those who refuse escorts without stating why. If there's an opportunity you think is safe to attend solo, always make sure someone knows where you are, who you are with, and how to contact that person.

A resourceful mercenary also scouts her location. Check Google Maps' street view to see if you're heading to a well-trafficked office building or a run-down trailer park.

When in doubt, put your safety first. You can always back out of a job—and you should do so if it makes you uncomfortable.

A professional doesn't participate in a shoot that will compromise her integrity. Photographers sometimes shoot on a location without getting permission from the owner. If you end up somewhere that makes you uncomfortable, you always have a right to leave. Claim allergies, an urgent phone call, or whatever you need—but it's okay to back out if something just doesn't feel right. Take your own car to each location, and keep your kit packed for a quick getaway.

A smart mercenary is extra wary of ads on Craigslist, especially if she prefers not to be involved in shoots with adult content. Sometimes ads are posted by harmless students, but there are a lot of people trying to make adult content. Look for jobs elsewhere—such as film commission websites, art school bulletin boards, or Model Mayhem (filter out 18+ posts). Do your research before meeting up with strangers. Don't let people take advantage of you because you are new. Trust your intuition; no opportunity is worth more than your safety.

Mission 6: Objective Summary

1. **Treat every job as seriously a paying job.** Handle yourself with the same professionalism as you would for paying clients—even if it's a trade job. Build the habits you'll need to be successful and prove to photographers that you can handle pro work.
2. **Become indispensible.** Make yourself an integral part of the team. Be fast, efficient, and humble. Lend a

hand when needed—even if the work falls outside of your job description.
3. **Leave a great impression.** Arrive early and leave when asked. When challenges arise, don't break a sweat. Stay calm and make your client's day better.

MISSION 7

The Payout

There's nothing like the feel of cold, hard cash. A professional may cherish her paydays, but she knows that she can't rest on her laurels. After a couple of jobs, you may start to realize that you need new makeup for the next shoot and your profits are still in the negative. This is when you have to shift your mentality from student to mercenary makeup artist. It's time to treat your hobby as a business.

Seek Professional Jobs

Even a talented mercenary struggles to find offers for paid work—at least until her reputation has spread. A great portfolio may get you many requests to trade your work for photos, but it takes time to bring in paying jobs. In the meantime, be selective with unpaid jobs. If a client seems good enough to net you future paying jobs, try working with him or her. However, be aware that unpaid work blocks out time that could be used for paying jobs. If the paying work is slow to come in, then this won't be an issue. Treat unpaid jobs professionally and honor your commitments—even if it means turning down a last-minute paying job. Remember, you'll gain more in the long run by working regularly and building your network, even if you have to turn down a job or two in the short term.

Value Your Time

A professional understands the value of her time and can charge $100 or more per hour. When you break down that rate—deducting taxes, supplies, and gas—it amounts to a lot less. That rate doesn't include time for commuting, setting up, cleaning up, and washing brushes. Makeup rates are also typically a series of one-time payments, whereas a full-time job is steady income.

A smart mercenary knows that a makeup business demands time above and beyond that for which her clients are willing to pay. There's the time to network, track down jobs, correspond with clients, and more. Makeup artistry can easily become as time-consuming as a full-time job. Keep your day job and pursue makeup as a side job. Benefits such as health insurance and retirement are harder to come by as a self-employed artist. You may reach a point where you make enough money to support yourself full-time, but it could take awhile. Don't let any trace of desperation show—it can sabotage your best impression and paint you as an amateur. Success is often a matter of persistence in this business, so don't lose hope if you can't afford to quit your day job.

Set Your Rates

A professional sets her rates long before her first job. To determine your rates, look to other artists in the area. If they don't post their rates, email them to inquire. You'll get more clients with lower rates, but you also might be underselling yourself. Higher rates tend to attract fewer people, but they are also a mark of an experienced artist. Look at how your portfolio compares to other professionals in your area, and set your prices accordingly. Lean towards lower rates until you gain more experience, but don't be afraid to raise them as you become more seasoned.

Draw up rates for a variety of situations. Are false lashes included for a bride? How about her bridesmaids? Offer packages for wedding parties or discount rates for extra headshot looks. Charge a fee for remote locations. The base charge for each service usually includes travel and set up, so offer discounts for additional clients or looks at the same location.

Get Paid

A smart mercenary counts the cash before she leaves. You might not want to be so obvert, but it's a good idea to be extra vigilant whenever money is being exchanged. Set up your payment methods in advance and inform your client what you accept so there will be no confusion. Do you take personal checks? If so, how will you handle a bounced check? Cash is the simplest method, but be sure to keep careful records for your taxes. Depositing cash into your business bank account on the day of the job creates a digital record that may make business accounting easier.

Some artists also accept credit cards through PayPal or reputable smart phone credit card readers such as Square. For little to no startup cost, you can accept payments online or instantly with a smart phone card reader. The main downside is that credit card transactions typically take a 3% fee from your payment. Credit card payments can also bring additional risks. For example, I had a photographer friend who had a rare situation where a client received her photos and then refused to pay—by getting her credit card company to dispute the charge. However, many artists feel that the convenience is worth the cost and potential risk. Check your local regulations for details on whether or not these types of services could work for your business.

For more on payment terms, see Sample Terms and Conditions in Mission 8: Bridal Makeup for Mercenaries.

Join a Team

A wise mercenary admits when a job is too big for her to handle alone. Large wedding parties are nearly impossible without at least one additional artist. Look for reputable artists in your area. Meet with them and draw up an agreement in writing so you'll be clear on how to split the money. Some artists may ask for a higher percentage if they book the job. Other artists might want to split the money down the middle. Who is responsible for the bride's makeup? Does one of you do foundations and prep while the other finishes each look? Whose kit do you use? If you carpool, who pays for gas? Work out these details ahead of time.

The truly dedicated may opt to work at a cosmetic counter or makeup store. You won't see a high payout per job, but you'll gain a lot of experience—often in a collaborative environment. An employee discount can make a kit much more affordable.

Mission 7: Objective Summary

1. **Actively pursue paying work.** Present yourself professionally online and in person. Look for postings and keep up with your network to hear about paying jobs.
2. **Determine your rates.** When job offers come your way, you want to be prepared with your rates. Find a balance between an attractive rate and one that will sustain your business.
3. **Recruit a partner.** If you can't make a job, to whom will you refer clients? Ideally, this person should also be someone you can call to help out on large jobs. Get your partnership terms drawn up in writing so there won't be any confusion.

MISSION 8

Bridal Makeup for Mercenaries

Bridal makeup will form a core part of your income as a mercenary makeup artist. If you can make a woman feel like a princess on her wedding day, she just might pay you like one. Bridal makeup is by far the largest and most accessible market. There is bridal makeup work in towns across the country—not just in big cities. If you want steady work in this industry, you must master bridal makeup and all that it entails.

Target Brides

A professional makes her services attractive to brides. Make sure your portfolio—or a sub-portfolio—focuses on your best bridal work. Make contacts with wedding venues, wedding photographers, and other professionals in the industry. List "bridal makeup" as one of your services on sites such as Yelp.com. For more ideas, see Mission 5: Marketing and Networking.

Correspond Promptly and Professionally

A professional responds to all job inquiries within 24 business hours. Bridal inquiries are business emails, so avoid casual language and emoticons. Reply from a computer, as opposed to a phone or tablet. You want to give the impression of a well-constructed, thoughtful reply—not just a "Yes, I'm available!" Reread before sending to catch any typos.

Emails can also help you get a sense of a bride's demeanor. Is she prompt, clear, and committed? Or does she constantly reschedule your appointment and take a week to respond? A professional interprets the cues and will gracefully back out if a client is more trouble than she's worth. Sometimes brides may ask for a service you don't yet offer, such as airbrushing. Other times, she might have a large party and you might not have a partner artist you can trust. Be clear if you can't accommodate her requests. If you do refuse a job, always include recommendations for other local artists.

Always remind your clients of appointments. When you set an appointment weeks or months in advance, it's easy for your client to forget. Send your client an email reminder the day before the appointment. Include the date, time, and location. This one simple email can save you misunderstandings or a wasted trip, and it gives you an email trail if you need to insist on payment for a missed appointment.

Showmanship is essential to inspiring confidence in the bride. Use a cheerful, professional tone to convey enthusiasm—even if you have to fake it. Stiff, formal emails can be misinterpreted as hostile. A bride is more likely to forgive eagerness than apathy.

Here is a sample reply to bridal availability queries:

Hi [BRIDE NAME],

Congratulations on your engagement! Thank you so much for your email. I would be happy to assist you on your wedding day.

I currently have availability on the morning of [DAY OF WEEK, DATE]. My rates are $X for you (including a trial run, usually 1-2 weeks before the wedding for the bride only), and $X each for your mother and sister. This comes to a total of $X if you wish to do all three. Application time is approximately 30 minutes per person, for a total of about 1.5 hours. If needed, I can be available at or before 7 a.m. for an additional $X fee. I can also work simultaneously with a hair stylist, if you are having one that morning as well.

Thank you for your interest and have a great week!

Best,
Kaylin

If the bride wants to book my services, I send this email:

Hi [BRIDE NAME],

I would be honored to be a part of your wedding day. I would like to arrive at your home by 7:30 a.m. on [DATE] to ensure that you are able to get to the venue on time. I will do your makeup before the rest of the bridal party, so you have plenty of time to dress and relax.

I have attached my Bridal Contract, which you can review at your convenience. Regarding payment, I require a 50% non-refundable deposit on the day of the trial run, which I typically schedule 2-3 weeks before the wedding. Are there any good dates or times for you in that window? Also, where is your home located?

If you have any ideas regarding the type of look you'd like on your big day, I'd love to hear them. Sometimes brides send me a few photos from the web or have some magazine clippings handy.

Thank you and I look forward to working with you!

Best,
Kaylin

The day before the trial run, I send this email:

Hi [BRIDE NAME],

I'm looking forward to meeting you for our trial run at [TIME] on [DAY] at [LOCATION] on [STREET NAME].

If you have any questions, I can be reached via email or cell: [INSERT PHONE NUMBER]. Have a great day!

Thanks,
Kaylin

If I refuse a job, I try to be courteous and helpful:

Congratulations on your engagement! Thank you so much for your email. Unfortunately, I am already booked that day and unable to take on additional appointments. I have included some other artists below that I recommend.

Thanks for your interest and have a great week!

Best,
Kaylin

Other Artists I recommend:
[PASTE LINKS TO LOCAL MAKEUP ARTIST WEBSITES HERE]

Insist on Trial Runs
A mercenary understands that bridal makeup has very different requirements than commercial shoots. You are applying makeup directly onto the client, many of whom have had little experience with professional makeup application. For this reason, do a trial run with wedding clients and try to avoid last-minute jobs.

When a professional arrives for a trial run, she should already understand the bride's vision. It can be anything from "rainbow peacock" to "something soft and natural." Always allow an hour for trial runs. Most brides want something very similar, but it often requires redoing the look before they are satisfied. This is why the trial run is an essential step to keeping a bride relaxed and happy on her wedding day.

Be sure to take before and after photos, including eyes open and eyes closed to show the full eye makeup application. Clients may even give you permission (in writing) to use them on your website. Use a face chart to keep track of each product used, so you can easily pull them ahead of time to re-create the look on the wedding day. In the rare event of an emergency, these notes and photos will easily allow a substitute artist recreate the same look on the wedding day.

Draw Up Bridal Contracts
A professional gets her bridal clients to sign a contract. Makeup artists typically reserve a date weeks or months in advance and may have to turn down other paid work on the same day. Bringing a bridal contract to the trial

run means fewer surprises on the wedding day—which is a very good thing.

Send the contract by email ahead of time and bring 2-3 printed copies to a trial run. When talking about contracts, don't let the bride sign the contract until the deposit amount is written down—you want the fees to be crystal clear. If a bride is taking a long time to book, tell her that you'd like to hold the day but you're getting other inquiries. A professional is never pushy, but knows how to gently nudge to book jobs.

A good contract contains all the basic information regarding the bride and her wedding, states the services included and the fee, and lists in clear terms the conditions of your agreement. Weddings can and do get cancelled, so a bride needs to know what will happen if it does. Be sure to list any additional fees. Important considerations include early call time fees and holiday fees, as well as parking fees, tolls, and other wedding-related expenses. For a sample contract, see www.kaylinskit.com.

My contract includes the following: bride's name, full address, and phone; date of contract, wedding date and time, wedding day contact, trial run date, location, and fee; wedding date time and location; itemized list of makeup applications (bride, bridal party and quantity, flower girls, add-on fees), bridal head count, travel fees, additional services, known allergies, deposit due on signing, balance due on wedding day, total due, and a list of additional services.

I have included sample terms and conditions below. Consult a lawyer after making your own contract, particularly if you want it to hold up in court. I have been lucky not to have many difficult clients, so I haven't had to enforce these terms and conditions. However, a professional is prepared to stand behind her contract and will enforce it if necessary.

SAMPLE TERMS AND CONDITIONS

A non-refundable deposit of 50% of all estimated fees is required on signing and holds your wedding date. The deposit is applied toward your final balance. By signing this contract, you are locking in the prices above, even if the rates increase before your wedding day. We accept cash, check, or PayPal only. Bride is responsible for any fees due to insufficient funds or other payment complications. A late fee of $10 per day will be assessed if the full balance is not paid by the day of the wedding. A final head count for makeup application is due 30 days prior to the wedding date. You will be billed by the final head count. No refund will be given for members of the Bridal Party who miss their appointment. The trial fee ($X) must be paid on the day of the trial.

No refunds on makeup services already applied. Cancellations made up to 48 hours before the wedding date are eligible for refunds for services not yet completed (minus the 50% non-refundable deposit). If a cancellation is made within 48 hours of the wedding date, you are responsible for the full amount of services in the agreed upon contract. The bride and members of the bridal party are responsible for disclosing their own allergies to makeup and/or products. [YOUR BUSINESS NAME] reserves the right to refuse service as necessary.

PREPARE STRATEGIES FOR CHALLENGING CLIENTS

You must learn how to handle even the most difficult clients. You may have heard rumors of sweet, kind-hearted women whose personalities crumble under the stress of a wedding. Often dubbed "bridezillas," these are usually just ordinary women who are having a rough time. If they treat you poorly, it usually isn't your fault.

I have had many wonderful brides, many of which probably wouldn't have even required a contract. However, there was one woman who was very particular about her makeup. She wanted a very soft, natural look and I redid it three times before she approved. I spent extra time at her trial run, but I sensed that she still wasn't quite happy. This bride didn't wear makeup normally and never quite seemed to feel natural in it. She called me up a few days after the trial run and asked that I refund her money. I calmly explained that she had paid the 50% deposit, almost all of which was for the trial run, which we had completed. She then demanded I refund the remaining $25 (50% deposit on another bridal party member) because she was cancelling.

This was a difficult situation, as she had signed a contract stating that the $25 deposit was non-refundable. When I mentioned this, she threatened to bring in her father, who was a lawyer. My strategy of being polite and courteous was no longer working. I knew that I could try to enforce the contract, but it was turning into an ugly and stressful situation. I chose to refund the $25, because it wasn't worth the trouble or risking my business' reputation.

When you encounter challenging clients, always be courteous and professional. If an email or call makes you upset, always take time to cool off before answering. "The customer is always right" adage is often true in the makeup industry. Consider the time and effort involved, and try to remedy the situation as quickly as possible. A professional knows when to swallow her pride for the sake of her business—even if she never made a mistake.

Expand Your Business

Mercenaries who want to make serious money from bridal makeup have to employ advanced strategies. Working solo can limit your opportunities, as you'll be unable to handle larger parties. Team up with another pro or take on an assistant to help with larger groups. See more about partnering in Mission 7: The Payout.

Ambitious mercenaries can also book more than one wedding per day. This works best if the weddings are spaced several hours apart. Be sure that you have adequate time to clean up, eat, drive between locations, and arrive 20-30 minutes early at the next location. If you won't have enough time to clean brushes, invest in a second (or even a third) set of brushes, particularly those that are hard to clean on site.

Putting it All Together: From Trial Run to Wedding Day

A professional has to keep a lot of steps in order, and it may seem complicated at first. Using my sister's wedding as an example, I've listed what it looks like to work with a bride to create her ideal look. This was a relatively small wedding and I was the only makeup artist, so the needs of your own jobs may vary.

One Week Before the Trial Run (Three Weeks Until the Wedding)

Discuss the bridal look with the client via phone or email. For example, my sister sent me some images of Kristen Bell and Emma Stone with red carpet makeup, which gave me an idea of the look she wanted. Choosing a celebrity with similar coloring can help a great deal in making a selection for a wedding day look.

The Day Before the Trial Run (Just Over Two Weeks Until the Wedding)

Email the bride a cheerful reminder with the trial run date, time, and location.

The Trial Run (Two Weeks Until the Wedding)

Wear flawless makeup and dress professionally. Have the bride review and sign your bridal contract. Run through the entire look with the client. Review images with client again (printed or on a tablet). Choose a target look (ours was a red-carpet image of Kristen Bell) and do your best re-creation on the client's face. Look for any large differences between your client and the celebrity, making sure to bring up anything that may turn out differently than your client expects before applying makeup. For example, if a client only gives you images of a warm-toned celebrity and they have a cool skin tone, let them know you will choose similar but different shades to better suit their complexion. Mention false lashes if you see them in the image and ask if your client wants this service.

After the initial application, be prepared to present a second option. With most of my bridal clients, I often remove the eye makeup and apply a second look. Even if all of your brides end up with the same look, the trial run is the time to indulge your client. Apply a gold foiled eye, black lipstick, or any other special request and let them decide for themselves.

Take notes and cell phone photos. Once you have settled on a look, take reference images (including one each with eyes open and eyes closed). Also, take notes regarding which products you used. I use face charts to keep track of the cosmetics. Collect the deposit before you leave.

THE NIGHT BEFORE
Set aside the bride's makeup, using your notes for reference. This ensures that you will at least have all of her makeup ready ahead of time, and won't have to dig through your kit to find any missing item.

WEDDING DAY, 7:30 A.M. (2.5 HOURS UNTIL THE WEDDING)
Leave for bridal venue. Load up your makeup kit and head to the venue (or, in some cases, a hotel or residence). Some wedding venues can be quite far from the city, so plan accordingly to arrive early. Wear flawless makeup. If the appointment is very early, it's better to wear no makeup than makeup that is poorly applied.

WEDDING DAY, 8 A.M. (2 HOURS UNTIL THE WEDDING)
Arrive at the venue and set up. Create a space to apply your makeup. Ideally, this should be somewhere peaceful where the bride and other members of the bridal party can relax. Natural light is important as well.

Wedding Day, 8:10 a.m. (Just under 2 hours until the wedding)

Apply the bride's makeup. Her makeup should be applied before anyone else's in the bridal party. Pay the most attention to the bride, even though her makeup should already be set aside. She needs to look flawless; the bridesmaids and other members of the party are less of a priority. You may be working simultaneously with a hair stylist.

Wedding Day, 8:45 a.m. (Just over 1 hour until the wedding)

Apply makeup for other members of the bridal party. This includes the mother of the bride, bridesmaid(s), flower girl, etc. For this wedding, I was only applying makeup to the bride and the mother of the bride, but allow 20-30 minutes per additional person. Adjust your estimates if you are skipping steps (only doing eyes, for example) or doing something complicated (such as applying individual lashes). Never book more than two hours of time on your own; if you need longer than this, hire a partner artist. At this point, the bride should be free to dress, get her hair styled, or relax.

Wedding Day, 9:15 a.m. (45 minutes until the wedding)

Complete final bride touch-ups. Do one last check, especially for powder and lip gloss. Make sure she has everything she needs. Remind her to carry her favorite lip gloss for touch-ups during the reception. Give her a cheap pack of mattifying papers to keep oil at bay.

Wedding Day, 9:30 a.m. (Half an Hour Until the Wedding)

Clean up and get out of the way. Leave well before the bride even thinks about walking down the aisle. Don't be the person holding up the wedding. Aim to finish 15 minutes before you think you want to be ready, in case the clients are running behind or there are other unforeseen circumstances.

Mission 8: Objective Summary

1. **Market to brides.** Find ways to reach out to brides. Feature bridal makeup prominently on your website. Try to get on vendor lists at wedding venues.
2. **Draw up a bridal contract.** Type up a contract and draw up your terms and conditions. Determine what types of services incur extra fees. See www.kaylinskit.com for a sample bridal contract.
3. **Set your bridal makeup policies.** Respond to emails from brides within 24 hours. Insist on trial runs. Don't work with a bride if you don't feel good about your interactions with them.

MISSION 9

Secret Techniques

An artist is shaped by those who train her. I learned from several other artists, each with his or her own style. While this is not a book on makeup techniques, I want to pass along some of the best advice from my seasoned mentors. Take or leave these tips, but continue experimenting to discover the techniques that will make your style all your own.

Use Your Hands

A professional may use disposables, brushes, and other tools, or she may be very hands-on. Clean hands are acceptable tools of the trade, provided your clients don't have severe allergies. I utilize the clean back of my hand as a "palette." I use disposable sponges for foundations, but hands to apply moisturizer or primer. Brushes are great for eye makeup, but fingers can help pull eyelids taut. I would find it hard to work without using my hands as tools. Some artists feel more connected to their clients by incorporating touch as part of the application.

If you choose to use your hands, be mindful of any pigments on them. You wouldn't want to mar your perfect foundation application with a black mascara streak, for example.

Primers Make a Professional

Whether or not you use primers as part of your everyday routine, they are an essential component of a professional application. Always use foundation primer and eye shadow primer. Each step in a professional's lengthy application process is there for a reason. From toning and moisturizing to using three products on lips, multiple layers set a professional application apart from everyday looks. Photographers, models, actors, and other clients depend on your work to last, and primers can help.

Foundations Are an Art

A trained professional knows that many women wear foundation that doesn't quite match their skin tone. This is often due to a number of factors, from applying foundation in artificial light to using the same foundation year round (despite skin lightening or tanning with the seasons). A professional will mix a custom foundation for her clients to ensure a perfect match. A shade that might pass in a dim restaurant might be obviously too yellow under studio lights. Work with a broad variety of clients with a range of skin tones, and soon you'll start to master the art of foundation matching.

Custom Matching Foundations

A professional can mix a custom foundation with mercenary efficiency. Before applying foundation to a client, look at their skin tone—ideally in natural light. Is it cool, neutral, warm, or somewhere in between? Is the tone fair, medium or deep? For a quick reference, hold up bottles to their faces to get a rough idea. Pick out two or three shades, and swipe each along your client's jawbone, from cheek to neck. If a shade blends in, that is generally a sign of a good match. If none are quite right, look closer. Is the client's skin tone between two shades (one is too dark and another too light)? Or is the discrepancy in the tone (too red or too yellow)? Mix a couple of shades together to balance the shade accordingly. Then test a strip of this foundation the same way. After some practice, you should be able to get a good match in no time.

Matching the Face or the Neck

Some clients have noticeably different tones between their faces and their necks. This often occurs from wearing sunscreen exclusively on the face or from skin conditions such as rosacea. In these cases, try and think about what would look best. If your client's face is noticeably lighter or redder than their neck and their neck appears a more natural tone, then you'll likely want to match the neck. You can apply foundation to the neck as well, but I generally only recommend this if there is some discoloration on the neck. The goal is to avoid making your client look as if he or she is wearing a mask.

I'll never forget when I first applied foundation to a client with rosacea. I took my time, mixing a foundation from my usual liquid plus a bit of concealer for more coverage. As her face was quite red, I chose the tone based on her neck. When the client's friend came in a few minutes later, she hardly recognized her. She was delighted to see her friend's best features on display—including her beautiful eyes and lips. The client herself was thrilled; she hadn't realized her own inner beauty. These are the moments that remind me why I love being a makeup artist.

SCARS, TATTOOS, AND OTHER ANOMALIES
A mercenary knows when to reach for the big guns. Some clients have scars, burns, or other skin conditions that require some special care. Your clients will typically disclose this information ahead of time, but they might not. Research color balancing techniques in books such as *About Face*. In a pinch, use a concealer like a cream foundation. If you have prior knowledge of the condition and the skin tone to match, stock your kit with a heavy-duty foundation from a brand such as Cinema Secrets. They offer full-coverage foundations and products for tattoo coverage as well. Keep in mind that you can charge a fee for special services such as tattoo covers. Another option for fuller coverage is airbrush makeup (see below).

AIRBRUSHING
Some professionals swear by airbrushes. They are a growing trend in the field, particularly in bridal makeup work. To learn airbrush makeup, take a course or workshop. Airbrush kits often are hundreds of dollars, and that doesn't always include the special airbrush makeup (usually foundation and blush). If there is a demand for airbrush makeup in your area, add it as a service once your business is profitable. Airbrush makeup is often applied for an additional fee. I have found great results from standard products and have felt that I can still get a light, natural look without airbrushing. If you plan to work high-end markets such as

Los Angeles and New York, airbrushing is more important to learn to stay competitive.

Start Soft

A professional gets her job right the first time. Sometimes, this means having some restraint. It can be difficult to remove extra blush or eye shadow without removing cosmetics layered beneath it. So start with a light makeup application, and then build to the coverage you need. The more you work with your cosmetics, the more familiar you will become with the coverage of each product. Tailor your applications to the needs of each project, and soon you'll be able to apply each cosmetic with mercenary efficiency.

If you're having trouble getting adequate coverage with a powder, apply it wet. For eye shadow, this is typically called "foiling." Spray a bit of water onto your brush, and then dip it into the powder. Gently dab it onto the eyelid to create a more intense, concentrated look. Powder concealer and powder blush can also be applied wet for different effects.

Eyebrows are for Shaving

Eyebrows can make or break a look. Keep a set of tweezers in your kit, but use them for splinters or shrapnel—never eyebrows. Tweezing eyebrows leaves redness that can detract from your application. If you run into a client with unruly brows, ask if you can use a small shaver to shape them. Use a battery-operated personal groomer, which is quick and painless. They are about the size of a pen and have a tiny blade about half an inch long.

Shaving allows you to quickly define a line without the potentially permanent effects of plucking.

Some makeup artists argue that eyebrow grooming isn't a makeup artist's responsibility. A mercenary without an esthetician's license or proper training should think twice before touching severely unruly brows. However, if you see some stray hairs or a unibrow, a shaver can provide a quick solution. State regulations regarding brow treatments may vary, so a smart mercenary should check to make sure brow shaving is in the clear.

Love Those Lashes
Mercenary Mascara

A professional doesn't bat an eye when it comes time to do her clients' mascara. To apply mascara with mercenary precision, take a disposable mascara wand and swipe it several times around your tube of mascara. Then have your clients keep their eyelids half-closed as you wiggle the wand gently from the roots of their lashes to the tips. Clients can even blink into the wand as you apply—just don't get the wand in their eye. Get plenty of mascara on your wand the first time. If you put a used wand back in your mascara, you will contaminate the entire tube. In the rare event that you need more mascara, use a new wand. Coat all the lashes—tops and bottoms—from inner corner to outer corner.

Curling lashes is simple for a professional. Instead of using one of those metal torture devices, opt for a heated lash curler. Curl after mascara has dried and keep a spare battery on hand. If you are applying false lashes, wait to curl until after the lashes have been applied.

Flawless False Lashes

A professional is also skilled in the art of false lashes. For brides, I prefer natural-looking lash strips. (Save the glitter, wild lengths, and sparkles for artistic looks.) Before applying, ask your client if they want false lashes. Some clients may have eyelash extensions, allergies to latex eyelash glue, or other special circumstances that you should take into account.

To apply a full lash strip, peel it off the packaging. Hold one end between each of your index fingers and thumbs. Wiggle the lash back and forth like a slinky or a caterpillar to loosen it. Then measure the lash strip on your client's eyelid. If it is too long, clip it with scissors (well away from your client's eyes). For a flirty touch, cut a full strip into half-strips to use on the outside edges of the eyes. You can use the smaller (beginning) half for a softer look or the longer (ending) half for a more dramatic look.

When the lash is the perfect length, apply a drop of lash glue to the end of a brush handle. Then run the glue along the lash strip in a very thin line. Wait a few seconds or until the glue appears tacky, not runny. Then apply the lash to the eyelid, using the end of a brush handle to help place it if necessary. Have your client keep their eye half-open to avoid gluing their eye shut. Glue the lash strip **just above** the lash line—not to the lashes. After the glue has dried, touch up the eyeliner if necessary (eyeliner goes on before lashes). Repeat with the second lash.

A professional can apply lashes in a flash—and keep her client smiling the whole time. Lashes can be daunting for brides and many other clients, so confidence is key. Practice applying false lashes on yourself until you are comfortable with the process.

Pair Creams with Powders

A resourceful mercenary knows how to get the most out of her cosmetics. Creams blend well together, but they often disappear quickly unless they are set with powder. Powder helps seal in creams and extends their wear. Use this two-part process in almost any application: liquid foundations beneath finishing powder, cream concealer beneath finishing powder, cream blush beneath powder blush, and cream eyeliner beneath powder liner (or matte eye shadow). When layered over a cream, powders can provide a matte, finished look that you can't achieve with creams or powders individually.

Breathe Carefully

If you need makeup that will hold up under the toughest conditions, specialized products may be in order. Apply them cautiously. Have clients exhale when applying white powders (such as silicone powders or HD finishing powders). This reduces inhalation of the product. When applying finishing sprays, both you and your client should hold your breath. Spray in an "X" shape, and then in a "T" shape.

Lips Need Touch-Ups

No matter how expertly a professional applies lip color, clients will inevitably need lip touch-ups. People have to eat and drink, so reduce wear on lip color by giving clients straws for drinks. When you won't be around to touch up lips, ask your clients to carry their favorite lip color and reapply after eating. This is especially useful for brides, who will want to eat, drink, and be merry at receptions.

Use an Eraser

A mercenary in training is going to make mistakes during her applications. If you discover that one of your cat eye wings is longer than the other, never fear. Dip a cotton swab in a bit of makeup remover, and swipe it along like an eraser. However, this technique has one main drawback: it removes the mistake and often everything beneath it, including eye shadow primer, foundation, and other important layers.

Fans Banish Fallout

Prepare for the possibility of eye shadow "fallout" on the under-eye area. Makeup artists use a couple of techniques to handle this. The first is dusting extra finishing powder beneath the eyes. Using a fan brush, swipe off the loose powder along with the fallout at the end. If you don't apply extra powder, you can also use the fan brush on just the fallout, but this technique is a little less effective.

If in Doubt, Toss It Out

A professional keeps a vigilant eye on her kit to ensure its freshness. If your makeup starts to separate, smell funny, change texture, turn colors, or otherwise seem suspicious, it's time to toss it out. General guidelines state that mascara lasts four to six months, liquid foundations and cream products last six to twelve months, lip products last up to two years, powders (such as finishing powders, blush, and eye shadows) and pencils (lip and eye) last two to three years. When it's time to trash your makeup, dump the product but recycle its container. Origins stores even offer a cosmetic container recycling program.

A Professional Application Process

The number of steps involved in a professional makeup application may seem daunting. Once you've gone through the process a few times, it should become second nature. It may still take you half an hour or longer, but if you organize your kit properly, it won't be nearly as complicated. Below is a sample of the process I use when applying makeup. For more on specific products and brushes, see Mission 3: Assemble Your Kit. For an application process checklist, go to www.kaylinskit.com.

Before You Begin

Wash hands and/or use hand sanitizer. Lay out a clean tissue or two for products, and make sure your kit is set out and ready for use.

Prep the Face

If the client has a full face of makeup, have them use a makeup remover towelette. Remove any traces of eye makeup with eye makeup remover. Apply witch hazel as a toner with a cotton ball, then apply a gentle moisturizer with hands or a foundation sponge. Apply lip balm with a lip brush, and then foundation primer with hands or a foundation sponge.

Foundation

Determine client's general skin tone and pick out 2-3 foundation shades. Test the shades, then mix a custom match with a plastic spatula in a paper nut cup. Test this shade, and then adjust if necessary. Once the right shade is mixed, apply using a foundation sponge. Make sure to extend the application slightly below the jaw line and blend well into the neck.

Eyebrows

Brush brows into place using an eyebrow comb or groomer. If brows are unruly, consider offering spot grooming with a shaver. Fill in any patches with an appropriate color of eye shadow or brow powder (or pencil). Brows should appear slightly darker than hair, but be sure to adjust for dyed hair. Use a small angled brush in short strokes to imitate hairs, or use a similar stroke with a pencil. When shading is complete, run a brow spoolie (or a disposable mascara wand) through unpetroleum jelly and gently brush into brows as a light brow gel.

Eyes

Apply eye shadow primer using a cotton swab. Layer base eye shadow color. Add deeper colors to crease or other areas based on eye shape and desired look. Pull eyelids taut when applying eye shadow and eyeliner for a cleaner look. Consider swiping a deeper shade to line the outer corners of the lower eye. Add any highlights, if necessary. Blend very well. Remove any eye shadow fallout with a fan brush.

If using a cream eyeliner, hold eyelid taut and sweep across eyelid with a narrow angled brush. Line the outer corners, then draw a line from the inner corners to meet it. Line below the eye last. Seal with matte eye shadow or eyeliner powder. Otherwise, use the appropriate eyeliner pencil and consider softening with an angled brush. Swipe disposable mascara wand around tube to pick up a lot of product, and then apply to lashes.

If using false lashes, measure and cut to appropriate length. Apply glue and wait until it becomes tacky. Apply lash gently just above lash line, and allow to dry. Make sure client keeps her eyes at least half-open throughout this process so her eyes won't get glued shut. Touch up eyeliner after lashes are in place, if necessary.

After mascara is dry, allow heated lash curler to warm up and then use to curl lashes. This is best done after false eyelashes are applied, if using lashes.

Concealer
Scoop concealer onto a palette or the back of your clean hand. Apply using a slick concealer brush. Use peach tones to balance blue under-eye circles, yellows to balance redness, etc. For blemish cover, tap brush gently over the blemish, concentrating on the lower (under) side. Also balance any additional redness, such as the nose or chin.

Finishing Powder
When the main face layers are complete, apply a layer of finishing powder with a powder brush. This may be a pigmented shade or a neutral (universal) shade. This will set the foundation, concealer, and other powders. Be sure to reach the under-eye area and the sides of the nose.

BLUSH, BRONZER, AND HIGHLIGHTER

If using a cream blush, blend into cheeks using hands or a foundation sponge; apply before finishing powder. If using powder blush, apply after finishing powder. Apply powder blush to cheeks, using a blush brush. Concentrate on the upper end of the apples of the cheeks, brushing upwards and outwards. If using bronzer, apply to the hollows of the cheeks, along the edges of the face, along the jaw line, and down the sides of the nose with a flat-topped brush. If using a lighter bronzer for a sun-kissed look, apply the same as highlighter: on the center of the forehead, down the front of the nose, on the tip of the chin, and across the tops of the cheeks. If using highlighter, also consider adding it beneath the eyebrow arch and just atop the center of the cupid's bow on the lips.

LIPS

After lip balm has soaked in, select a lip color. Start with a layer of an appropriate lip liner (typically nude to match the client's lips or red if using a red lipstick). Have the client smile to keep lips taut. Line lips and fill them in with liner as well. If using lipstick, brush on a quick layer with a lip brush. Top with lip gloss in an appropriate shade.

FINAL TOUCHES

When the look is complete, allow the client to review it in your hand mirror. Once approved by client or person in charge, apply setting spray, if using. If this is a look you will recreate, record the products used on a face chart and take quick photos for documentation. Then clean all brushes, sanitize makeup, and sharpen sanitized pencils before using on your next client. If you only have one client, handle the clean-up process after you've left.

Touch-Ups

After an application is complete, the client may require touch-ups to the lips as well as powder to prevent oiliness. If you can stay with the client, keep their lip color handy. Apply a silicone or universal finishing powder for touch-ups to avoid the cakey look of layered pigmented powders. If you can't stay with the client, have them keep their favorite lip color handy. Suggest they use a powder from time to time or leave a packet of cheap mattifying papers with them.

Mission 9: Objective Summary

1. **Refine your technique.** Seek out pro tips to find new ways to streamline the application process. Add new looks to your repertoire.
2. **Practice any weaknesses.** If you struggle with false eyelashes, practice applying them on yourself until you could practically do it in your sleep. Look up tips for any trouble areas in your applications, such as covering blemishes or applying bronzer.
3. **Fall into a routine.** Habits make the application process much simpler. Follow the same order and you're less likely to forget a step. See www.kaylinskit.com for an application process checklist.

MISSION 10

Set Your Aim High

Once you're a veteran mercenary, you'll have earned the right to bigger and better opportunities. If you're making plenty to support yourself and find the mercenary lifestyle unfulfilling, there are other lifestyles available to makeup artists. It may be time to become a highly-specialized professional and pursue your ideal career.

Set Your Aim

Upgrade Your Portfolio

A professional's portfolio should reflect her best work. Makeup trends change, so don't let your portfolio grow stale. The content may also need a shift if you're going to aim for national markets. Bridal photos you took with an amateur photographer might be great for bridal business, but they won't impress major magazine editors. Start copying amazing looks from the best of the best artists, and use these to develop your own style. Look for inspiration from artists such as Kevyn Aucoin, Scott Barnes, and Topolino.

A professional also has a collection of tear sheets. These coveted items are excerpts from magazines and other printed outlets—which contain your credited makeup work. Your first sheets might be from local or regional magazines, so try to work your way up to bigger and better outlets.

Get a Flexible Day Job

If mercenary makeup work isn't enough to support you, seek out a side job that will give you more time to focus on your makeup dreams. An ideal role for a mercenary is a stay-at-home, flexible hours job, such as graphic design, web design, data entry, or customer service. Even if makeup work isn't consistent, a flexible job will give you maximum availability for makeup jobs.

Attend Workshops

A professional is constantly learning. Gain new skills or brush up on old ones by attending workshops. Generally, shorter-term workshops will provide the most bang for your buck. Costs and locations can vary greatly. Check out workshops from Last Looks, MAC Pro Stores, Dinair, and others. IMATS (International Make-up Artist Tradeshow) also offers workshops.

Apprentice to a True Master

You will learn the most from true veterans—not instructors. Seek out those who are doing what you want to do and try to become their apprentice. Find people in your area, or look up artists on IMDb. An ideal apprenticeship offers experience on set—alongside the master artist and in the trenches. This may feel like a step back initially, but watch the master carefully. You'll pick up priceless tips through observation alone.

Network at National Shows

You might find local opportunities too limiting. A large convention or tradeshow can be a great way to connect with other professionals. One of the most respected events for pro makeup artists is the International Makeup Artist Tradeshow, or IMATS. Hosted by Make-up Artist Magazine, this event is a great way to connect with working makeup artists. There are demos and workshops, providing plenty of opportunities to network and learn from other artists. Another highlight of the show is the makeup vendors, who often offer greats discounts on tempting items for your kit. If you plan to travel for IMATS, reviewers recommend the Los Angeles show for the biggest and best experience in the U.S.

Shift Into High Gear
Get Representation

A seasoned professional should seek out representation for the best opportunities. Magazine photo shoots for national magazines and other exclusive jobs may be nearly impossible to get without an agent. Ideally, you would get an agent through contacts you make with an apprenticeship or other networking opportunity. For inspiration, look up Cloutier and Jedroot for a roster of some of the best working makeup artists.

Keep Your Target in Sight

When a professional hones in on her specialty, she must pursue it single-mindedly if she wants to succeed. The time for a diverse, mercenary approach is over. Choose a path and find out how deep the rabbit hole goes. Which career do you dream of pursuing?

Fashion – Typically based in New York or other fashion centers, these artists are responsible for bringing a fashion designer's or editor's vision to life. Makeup is often cutting-edge, colorful, and unique. This field has some of the greatest opportunities for creative looks.

Celebrity – From red-carpet events to celebrity magazine features, these makeup artists often become famous after gaining the trust of one or more celebrities. Some celebrities even bring makeup artist along to help them with makeup for movie premieres and other events. Makeup tends to range from natural to smoldering red carpet looks, with occasional high fashion work as well.

Entrepreneur – Some artists are obsessed with cosmetics, but not as interested in working with clients. If you know exactly what you want in each product but are having trouble finding it, entrepreneurship may be for you. Start your own makeup line and you can determine the formulations, shades, and prices. Some artists also consult for makeup lines, providing feedback and input on new products, without the financial investment.

MISSION 10: OBJECTIVE SUMMARY

1. **Set your sights on a specific career.** Allow yourself to dream big. Pursuing a career in a highly competitive makeup field is a big risk, but it can also be very rewarding.
2. **Get specialized training.** Look outside your region for classes and workshops in niche fields. Weigh the costs and benefits of traveling or moving to learn these specialized skills.
3. **Find a master.** Get your foot in the door by serving as an apprentice to an artist in your desired field. Humbly offer your services and observe the master at work.

DOSSIER

MERCENARY RESOURCES

Below is a list of resources found throughout the book's missions (with a few additions). They are arranged roughly in the order in which they are mentioned. This section focuses on U.S.-based resources, but many of them are applicable to artists in other countries as well. For clickable links and downloadable bonuses, check out www.kaylinskit.com.

BOOKS
Face Forward, by Kevyn Aucoin
Making Faces, by Kevyn Aucoin
Bobbi Brown Makeup Manual, by Bobbi Brown
Makeup Makeovers, by Robert Jones
About Face, by Scott Barnes
The 4-Hour Workweek, by Timothy Ferriss
The $100 Startup, by Chris Guillebeau
The 22 Immutable Laws of Marketing, by Al Ries and Jack Trout
NOLO's Small Business Start-Up Kit, by Peri Pakroo
How to Win Friends and Influence People, by Dale Carnegie

BEAUTY SCHOOL RESOURCES
NACCAS
naccas.org
Habia
www.habia.org
Aveda Institute
www.avedainstitutesbb.com

BEAUTY SCHOOL RESOURCES (CONT.)
Baldwin Beauty School
www.baldwinbeautyschools.com
Paul Mitchell – The School
www.paulmitchelltheschool.com
Beauty Schools Directory
www.beautyschoolsdirectory.com

BUSINESS LINKS
SCORE
www.score.org
U.S. Small Business Administration
www.sba.gov

KIT RESOURCES
MAKEUP BRAND RESOURCES
PETA
features.peta.org/cruelty-free-company-search/index.aspx
Leaping Bunny
www.leapingbunny.org
Environmental Working Group's Skin Deep database
ewg.org/skindeep

KIT RESOURCES (CONT.)

Note: "MUA Discount" refers to brands which offer a makeup artist discount (see Mission 3: Assemble Your Kit).

MAKEUP BRANDS AND TOP PRODUCTS

100% Pure
Lipstick, blush, and bronzer
www.100percentpure.com

Afterglow Cosmetics (MUA Discount)
White finishing powder
www.afterglowcosmetics.com

Alima Pure
Powder foundations in a wide color range
www.alimapure.com

Beauty Without Cruelty
Waterproof mascara, makeup remover, and moisturizers
www.beautywithoutcruelty.com

Cinema Secrets
Foundation for tattoo coverage
www.cinemasecrets.com

Crazy Rumors
Lip balms and tinted lip balms
crazyrumors.com

DeVita
Cream foundations and pressed powder eye shadows
devitaskincare.com

Ecco Bella
Liquid foundation, eye shadow (refills), powder eyeliner, and bronzer
www.eccobella.com

Eyes Lips Face (E.L.F.)
Mattifying papers, eye shadow primer, cheap false eyelashes, and other budget cosmetics
www.eyeslipsface.com

MAKEUP BRANDS AND TOP PRODUCTS (CONT.)

Gabriel Cosmetics/Zuzu Luxe (MUA Discount)
Liquid foundations, pressed powders, pressed eye shadows, eyeliner, pressed powder blush, lipstick, and lip liner
www.gabrielcosmeticsinc.com

Glo Minerals
Concealers
www.gloprofessional.com

Haut Minerals
Waterproof foundation
hautcosmetics.ca

Jane Iredale (MUA Discount)
Eyeliner, lip liner, eye shadows, pressed powders, and brush cleaner
janeiredale.com

Josie Maran
Moisturizers and eye shadow
www.josiemarancosmetics.com

Korres (MUA Discount)
Foundation primer, eye shadow primer, lip butter, and lip gloss
korresusa.com

Kryolan
Special effects and bruise palettes
us.kryolan.com

Manic Panic
Unusual lipstick colors (including black)
www.manicpanic.biz

Mehron
Special effects, spirit gum, face paints, and Halloween makeup
www.mehron.com

NVEY Eco
Pressed powder eye shadow, and pressed powder eyeliner
www.nveymakeup.com

NYX (MUA Discount)
Eyeliner, lip liner, and eye shadows
www.nyxcosmetics.com

Makeup Brands and Top Products (cont.)

Obsessive Compulsive Cosmetics (MUA Discount)
Eyeliner, lip tars, glitters, and color creams
occmakeup.com

Pacifica
Lip gloss
www.pacificaperfume.com

Physician's Formula (Organic Wear line)
Mascara and bargain cosmetics (liquid foundations, pressed powders, pressed powder blush, pressed powder bronzer, etc.)
www.physiciansformula.com

Tarte Cosmetics
Mascara, water-resistant cosmetics, cream eyeliner, and pencil eyeliner
tartecosmetics.com

Urban Decay (MUA Discount)
Eye shadow primer, false lashes, and setting spray
www.urbandecay.com

Makeup Reviews and Recommendations

Kaylin's Kit
www.kaylinskit.com

Brushes

Alima Pure
www.alimapure.com

bdellium Tools (MUA Discount)
bdelliumtools.com

Crown Brush
www.crownbrush.com

EcoTools (false lashes as well)
www.eco-tools.com

E.L.F. (for budget items and false lashes)
www.eyeslipsface.com

Nail Polish

Acquarella
acquarella.com

No Miss
www.nomiss.com

Rainbow Honey
www.rainbowhoney.com

Other Items

Beauty So Clean
www.beautysoclean.com

The Brush Guard
thebrushguard.com

Dinair Airbrushes
www.airbrushmakeup.com

Z Palette
zpalette.com

Zuca Pro Bag (MUA Discount)
www.zuca.com

Makeup Specialty Stores

Alcone (MUA Discount)
www.alconeco.com

Camera Ready Cosmetics (MUA Discount)
camerareadycosmetics.com

Naimie's Beauty Center (MUA Discount)
www.naimies.com

Sally Beauty Supply
Mascara wands, etc.
www.sallybeauty.com

Recycling Makeup

Origins Recycling Program
www.origins.com/cms/recycling_program/index.tmpl

Marketing and Networking

Portfolio Building
Model Mayhem
www.modelmayhem.com

Websites
Wix
www.wix.com
Blogger
www.blogger.com
Wordpress
wordpress.com
Elance
www.elance.com

Social Media
Facebook
www.facebook.com
Twitter
twitter.com
Instagram
instagram.com
LinkedIn
www.linkedin.com

Networking
Meetup
www.meetup.com
Wedding Wire
www.weddingwire.com
Yelp
biz.yelp.com
Google Places
www.google.com/mybusiness
Punchbowl (digital greeting cards)
www.punchbowl.com

Business Cards
Moo.com
us.moo.com

Business Cards (cont.)
Taste of Ink
tasteofink.com

Payments
PayPal
www.paypal.com
Square
squareup.com

Contracts
Please see www.kaylinskit.com for sample contracts.

Workshops
Dinair
www.airbrushmakeup.com
IMATS
www.imats.net
Last Looks
www.lastlooksmakeup.com
MAC Pro Stores
www.maccosmetics.com/macpro

Makeup Masters
Kevyn Aucoin
www.kevynaucoin.com
Scott Barnes
scottbarnes.com
Topolino
callisteagency.com/make-up/topolino
IMDb (Internet Movie Database)
www.imdb.com

Makeup Agencies
Cloutier Remix
cloutierremix.com
Jedroot
www.jedroot.com

About the Author

Kaylin Johnson is an eco-friendly makeup artist and consultant based in Austin, Texas. Her blog, Kaylin's Kit, features hundreds of makeup tips, articles, and product reviews. She has been featured in magazines and on sites such as Shape.com and Girlie Girl Army. She has also developed video tutorials for Rejuva Minerals and Tyra Banks' Typef.com. Kaylin enjoys working with a variety of clients, from actors and actresses to models and brides. In her spare time, she can often be found cooking vegan food, playing video games, or practicing knockout dance moves.